High-Throughput Formulation Development of Biopharmaceuticals

Related titles

Process Validation for the Production of Biopharmaceuticals
(ISBN 978-1-90756-864-0)

Woodhead Publishing Series
in Biomedicine: Number 69

High-Throughput Formulation Development of Biopharmaceuticals

Practical Guide to Methods and Applications

Vladimir I. Razinkov
Gerd R. Kleemann

ELSEVIER

AMSTERDAM • BOSTON • HEIDELBERG • LONDON
NEW YORK • OXFORD • PARIS • SAN DIEGO
SAN FRANCISCO • SINGAPORE • SYDNEY • TOKYO

Woodhead Publishing is an imprint of Elsevier

WP WOODHEAD PUBLISHING

Woodhead Publishing is an imprint of Elsevier
The Officers' Mess Business Centre, Royston Road, Duxford, CB22 4QH, United Kingdom
50 Hampshire Street, 5th Floor, Cambridge, MA 02139, United States
The Boulevard, Langford Lane, Kidlington, OX5 1GB, United Kingdom

British Library Cataloguing-in-Publication Data
A catalogue record for this book is available from the British Library

Library of Congress Cataloging-in-Publication Data
A catalog record for this book is available from the Library of Congress

ISBN: 978-1-907568-63-3 (print)
ISBN: 978-1-908818-76-8 (online)

For information on all Woodhead Publishing visit our website at https://www.elsevier.com

Publisher: Mica Haley
Acquisition Editor: Glyn Jones
Editorial Project Manager: Anna Valutkevich
Production Project Manager: Omer Mukthar
Designer: Mark Rogers

Typeset by MPS Limited, Chennai, India

Contents

About the authors

Vladimir I. Razinkov is a principal scientist in the Department of Drug Product Formulation Technologies, Amgen Inc., Thousand Oaks, California, USA.

Gerd R. Kleemann is a scientific director in the Department of Digital Integration and Predictive Technologies, Amgen Inc., Thousand Oaks, California, USA.

High-throughput methodology in biopharmaceutical formulation development

1

To this day, the Biopharmaceutical industry is struggling to fulfill its promise. Although about 30 years old, drugs are not developed notably faster, cheaper, or with better understood benefit and risk profiles. On the other hand, the number of automated high-throughput methodologies available for sample preparation, forced-degradation applications, and physicochemical analytics of proteins has increased dramatically over the last decade. Some of those methods were adopted from the development of small molecule pharmaceuticals and some methods have become high throughput with the help of increasing sensitivity and miniaturization of analytical instrumentation, and most importantly a higher level of automation. In light of internal and external pressures to reduce the cost of drug development and to stay competitive in an increasingly crowded marketplace, automation is becoming critical as a mechanism to lower the cost of research and development by liberating scientists from routine tasks.

The process of high-throughput formulation screening can be divided into several steps: design of experiment, sample preparation, stress assays for accelerated degradation studies, analytical methods, and data analysis (see Fig. 1.1). Each procedure can be developed separately, but ideally, for a workflow to be seamless, the transfer of samples and data between the different experimental workflows needs to be automated. The most important part of such a workflow is the information structure. For data to be comparable and easily transferrable between different studies, the methods and assays used in formulation studies have to be standardized (i.e., platform methods) with the same set of instrument and assay parameters (e.g., resolution, sensitivity, etc.). The experimental design takes into account the range of measured values for each study to avoid data gaps and unnecessary data redundancy. The lack of appropriate alignment between studies and the lack of assay and data standards is a common problem in formulation development. More than often, head-to-head comparisons of study data are compromised because the study, assay, and data parameters are not aligned and will not allow a direct correlation of output values across development studies and products. For example, if the drug development was interrupted for financial or strategic reasons, and then the candidate was reintroduced into the development cycle, the methods and analytical assays for formulation development used before may be outdated, different, and incompatible with new methodologies introduced after the reentry of the drug. Legacy drugs, inherited from a company merger or acquisition, are another example that illustrates the difficulty of processing incomplete or incompatible data sets. The gap in the data generated and obtained from the development by

High-Throughput Formulation Development of Biopharmaceuticals. DOI: http://dx.doi.org/10.1016/B978-1-907568-63-3.00001-3

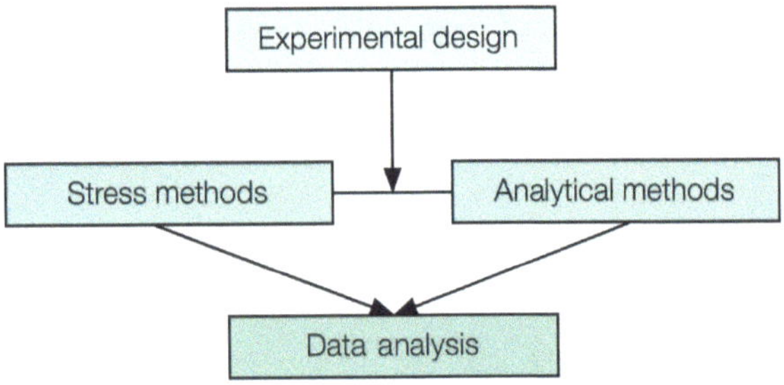

Figure 1.1 General steps of a high-throughput formulation screening workflow.

acquired companies can be significant and often requires large numbers of resources to appropriately complement or complete these insufficient data sets.

The "Quality by Design" (QbD) concept, implemented by the US Food and Drug Administration (FDA), has become the norm for the biopharmaceutical industry to develop processes that consistently produce products with quality attributes that meet the desired clinical performance parameters for clinical safety and efficacy [1].

In formulation development, the QbD concept is applied to understand the relationship between a process and a product's critical quality attributes (CQA), as well as the correlation between CQA and a product's clinical properties. The purpose of formulation studies is to establish these correlations and to find the relationships between input factors (e.g., solution compositions, stress conditions, time points, etc.) and analytical output or result data from various analytical experiments. The initial selection of input variables and the methods and assays to obtain output parameters generally relies on statistical applications like the approaches based on the "Design of Experiments" (DOE) methodology. DOE help formulation scientists to not only strategically plan and execute formulation studies, but most importantly, based on the analysis and interpretation of controlled test data, to evaluate the factors that control the value of a parameter or group of parameters. There are many examples of studies that follow the DOE-based methodology to establish a formulation design space [2,3]. DOE principles were applied in the study of the formation of mannitol hemihydrate in biopharmaceutical formulations [4]. To systematically investigate the destabilizing effect of mannitol hemihydrate on protein formulations, the authors used a composite face-centered study design, which included solid content, protein concentration, protein type, and mannitol/sucrose ratios as the formulation parameters of interest. Also, annealing as a process parameter was added to a full factorial mixed design. The DOE resulted in models with a high goodness of fit and prediction for different proteins. The addition of the process parameter annealing produced the same quality model. High protein concentration, low relative mannitol content, and annealing at low temperature were statistically significant factors to enhance mannitol hemihydrate formation. Additional case studies will be discussed in later chapters of this book.

During the experimental design stage, all available information about a molecule or formulation should be used to build a study strategy that enables the development of a formulation design space that controls CQA and stability acceptance criteria.

Sometimes two or more iterative studies are necessary to narrow down a study's input and output parameters to a design space that provides acceptable control and robustness. For example, a pH range from 3.0 to 8.0 with intervals of 0.5 between pH values may be tested first and then followed up by a study with a narrower pH range to create higher resolution around the most stability providing pH value (e.g., pH 4.5–5.5 with higher resolution pH intervals of 0.1). During the later stages of formulation development, robustness studies are necessary to demonstrate that slight deviations from the formulation target parameters will not negatively affect the drug product CQA. The deviations may include variability in excipient and protein concentration, fluctuations in temperature or moisture values for lyophilized formulations. Other parameters critical to product quality could be included in robustness studies (e.g., variation in container properties, shipping parameters, supply chain procedures, etc.). A strong statistical approach is required to evaluate the analytical results of the output parameters, particularly if differences in experimental data are small.

To increase efficiencies, create time savings, and relieve scientists from routine operating steps, the planning of formulation studies should also consider the process of sample handling and transfer from preparation to stress stations (i.e., stress-inducing assays that are stability indicating and differentiating) and analytical instruments. Integrating plate, vial, or syringe handling systems into an end-to-end experimental workflow would enable the automation of a significant number of processing steps of DOE-type formulation development studies.

The most common platform for handling large numbers of samples is the multi-well plate. Many liquid-handling systems, stress-inducing and analytical methods can accommodate multi-well plates for the analysis of a large variety of formulation parameters and sample volumes. The number of wells per plate and geometry of plates provide flexibility for tailoring the plate-design appropriately to study designs, as well as assay and analytical methods requirements. Most importantly, the automation of transfer of liquids and plates makes it possible to connect all operating steps of a high-throughput process. The creation of a consistent and seamless methodology with adjustable modules enables the interfacing for all the operating procedures starting from the mixing of formulation components to the placing of samples into analytical instruments for parallel analysis by a large variety of analytical characterization methods and technologies. Moving plates from pipetting or mixing platforms to chromatographic, spectroscopic, or other type of analytical instrumentation, requires a great deal of mechanical alignment, robotic capabilities, as well as software control and synchronization. Many manufacturing companies create and integrate their own line of detection and measurement instruments into their own sample handling stations. Those companies are also working in close collaboration with manufacturers of analytical technologies to synchronize the control of their software and hardware. For example, Tecan Group AG (Männedorf, Switzerland), the maker of liquid-handling workstations, has built-in spectrometers, which can handle multi-well plates and perform measurements under the control of the same instrument software that controls the automated liquid and sample handling capabilities of the workstation [5]. Tecan is also collaborating with other parties such as Wyatt Technology (Santa Barbara, California), a manufacturer of plate readers for light-scattering measurements, and

Tecan has built interfaces that allow seamless integration of Wyatt's plate readers into the Tecan technology platform. Wyatt Technology is also working with Agilent Technologies (Santa Clara, California) and Waters Corporation (Milford, Massachusetts) on in-line integration of chromatography-based separation with light-scattering detectors. Another company, Freeslate, Inc. (Sunnyvale, California), offers configurable, robotic laboratory automation systems that provide an integrated suite of automated formulation screening hardware and software that is able to combine liquid dispense and controlled heating/cooling/mixing with high-throughput capabilities for pH measurement, viscosity measurement, and visual inspection/particle counting. Combined with Freeslate's Lab Execution and Analysis (LEA) software, the system offers control and data integration extensions for a range of third party analytics including dynamic light scattering (DLS), ultraviolet/visible (UV/Vis) spectroscopy, capillary isoelectric focusing (cIEF), capillary SDS-PAGE (CE-SDS), high-performance liquid chromatography (HPLC), ultra-performance liquid chromatography (UPLC), etc. [6]. The system includes modules for high-throughput particle, turbidity, and color measurements. Separate incubation thermostats and components for different stress applications can be added. To create seamless workflows between study design and analytical analysis, computer software can enable the integration of DOE algorithms with instrumental control functions. Tecan Group AG has developed its own control software platform to translate DOE study setups, written with the statistical software JMP (SAS, Cary, North Carolina), into program scripts for the automated preparation of solutions on the Tecan workstations. These integrated and automated workflows create great efficiencies and time savings, especially for studies with large sample sizes or for batch studies that investigate large numbers of molecules or molecule candidates simultaneously. To achieve high accuracy and precision of automated high-throughput assays it is necessary to understand the exact contribution of each component to the system. Accuracy is a characteristic of how close a measured value is to its actual value. Therefore, accuracy of an assay is highly dependent on the performance of the analytical instruments in use, specifically the measurement components. Precision is a measurement of how close the measured values are to each other. Precision can be a function of reproducibility and sample size. Those parameters depend on specification of the automation components and the experimental design.

The different analytical methodologies that are applied for comprehensive analysis of product attributes produce massive data sets with a variety of different data formats. In general, each instrument has its own control and analysis software for running the instrument, processing of raw data, and report creation. Therefore, for complex, automated high-throughput experimental designs, the data analysis becomes the bottleneck rather than the execution of the sample preparation and analysis. For example, a peptide mapping analysis by high-performance liquid chromatography in conjunction with mass spectrometric analysis (HPLC-MS) can take less than 30 minutes. The data analysis, however, takes significantly more time to translate the "ion intensity versus m/z" plot of each mass spectrum into an actual protein sequence. Furthermore, for certain types of analysis additional steps, preceding the actual data analysis, need to be performed to prepare raw data for analysis by third party analysis programs (JMP,

SAS, R, etc.). These programs for statistical analysis often require data sets being ordered or structured in specific table or matrix formats. Proper data templates for exporting into third party data analysis programs are especially critical for multivariate analysis of complex data sets.

Many instruments and methods in high-throughput study formats have been used in the pharmaceutical and biopharmaceutical industry in the last two decades. Individual analytical methods such as UV spectroscopy [7], fluorescence, Fourier transform infrared (FTIR) spectroscopy [8], light scattering, calorimetry [9], and others have already been applied in different fields of drug development [10–13]. In the past, techniques with high-throughput capabilities have been used along with low-throughput methods as part of characterization studies. More recently, this combination of high-throughput with low-throughput technologies has also been applied for higher throughput formulation screening studies. In these particular cases the screening was focused on just a few important parameters and their analysis produced formulation recommendations based on the characterization of only one or two degradation pathways [14].

Integration of several methods into one characterization process to study a molecule's formulation design space not only helps with developing an understanding of stability providing parameters but also provides a greater understanding of the underlying degradation mechanisms. With increasing data sets the possibility to predict the stabilizing effects of formulation components becomes a reasonable possibility. Automation eliminates variability introduced by analysts and increases reproducibility of sample handling and in turn creates greater precision and accuracy in data analysis. Automated procedures also make it easy to detect outliers and instrumental errors. A good example of an automated formulation screening system is the robotic system and high-throughput laboratory (HTL) described by the scientists from Novartis (Basel, Switzerland) [15]. Their HTL platform is comprised of several analytical methods, developed for high-throughput analytics that are fully integrated into an automated laboratory to screen up to 500 antibody formulations at a time. Sample preparation was fully automated and was based on the microplate format. The data obtained by the high-throughput system were compared to the results generated by traditional approaches. Barcodes were used to track the different formulations and molecules. The different data formats, generated by the different analytical systems, were sorted and converted for analysis into a Spotfire (TIBCO, Inc., Palo Alto, California) compatible format. In this work, the high-throughput methods are limited to the techniques used for sample preparation and handling. Hence, opportunity exists to further accelerate the execution of formulation studies by developing and integrating analytical methodologies with high-throughput capabilities. It is becoming more of a general practice to not limit high-throughput technologies only to the area of sample preparation and handling but also to develop high-throughput analytical techniques and methodologies to further increase efficiencies and time savings in formulation development. In fact, combined automation of sample preparation, sample treatment, and measurement would make formulation development more time efficient and less costly.

High-throughput methods not only accelerate the process of finding the best formulation for a selected drug candidate or the best candidate for a specific formulation

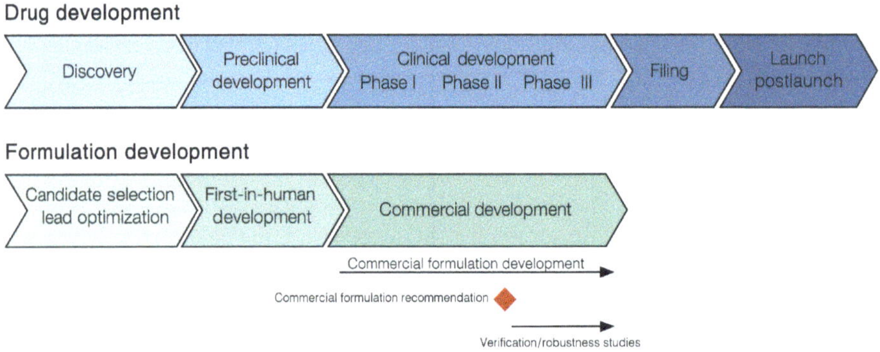

Figure 1.2 The stages of formulation development in a drug development process.

(i.e., platform formulation), but also collect information faster and more comprehensively. High-throughput methods also gather information and data sets that facilitate the development of models that may forecast protein stability with greater accuracy. A typical drug development process in the biopharmaceutical industry, which includes formulation development and involves several development phases, is shown in Fig. 1.2. Early phase formulation screening in support of either early candidate or formulation selection becomes feasible if an automated high-throughput process for sample preparation, sample handling, and sample analysis is available. In these early stages of development, the number of molecule candidates that need to be evaluated limits the variety of formulation conditions. Even, with the most automated and sophisticated high-throughput process, there is a limit of how many candidates can be assessed. Hence, the number of formulation conditions should be limited and stability indicating for the most critical stability attributes; often not more than one or two parameters (e.g., pH and a single storage temperature that are stability indicating and differentiating). This also holds true for the analytical methods, which should be wisely chosen in regard to their appropriateness to detect differences in the critical product attributes to enable the elimination of molecules with the least favorable stability properties. A smaller number of candidates allows formulation scientists to include more analytical methods and to expand the number of formulation parameters, which helps to develop a more comprehensive understanding of a product's critical product attributes and its formulation design space.

During the next phases of development (i.e., preformulation screening and manufacturability assessment), it is important to be able to rank the molecules and formulations rather than to eliminate the least stable ones. The ranking of molecule candidates and formulations becomes critical when factors other than those that determine product stability have the priority to determine the lead candidate (e.g., bioactivity, half-life, manufacturability, etc.). On the other hand, the evaluation of an expanded formulation space provides the opportunity to apply additional stress conditions (i.e., in the form of pH, temperature, ionic strength, etc.) to produce differentiating criteria for candidates that are otherwise equal in their stability profile. Also, at that stage of development there is an opportunity to simulate manufacturing, purification, and storage processes the drug product will encounter during downstream processes. The assessment of drug candidates by simulated conditions is called molecule or manufacturability assessment. High-throughput methodologies are very helpful in the screenings of multiple formulations exposed to various simulated conditions and the results of formulation screenings are used to create a stability profile in a multidimensional space of characterization parameters. Stability profiles can be compared between different drug candidates and predictions about stability properties can be made based on statistical analysis of high-throughput data. We will describe the methods of analysis in Chapter 5, High-throughput formulation development of biopharmaceuticals: practical guide to methods and applications.

As drug development has become a longer process and the number of new drug approvals has declined in the last decade, the pharmaceutical and biopharmaceutical industry has been under pressure to find new innovative ways to bring medicines into the market faster and with greater probability of success. The low success rates for drugs entering the preclinical and early clinical stage are among other things due to a lack of efficacy and toxicity data, poor absorption, distribution, metabolism, and elimination (ADME) properties, commercial interest and market competition. On the other hand, formulation and drug delivery strategies exist that better address the physicochemical properties that are critical for improved ADME and overall product stability properties [16].

It is desirable to identify the molecule candidate and formulation composition with the most favorable properties as early as possible. Unfortunately, the reality is that at the early stages of development the assessment of stability, manufacturability, and ADME properties depends on a selection process that requires the screening of a large variety of molecule candidates, formulation compositions, and the combination of the two. To facilitate screening of sample sizes that big, the use of 96-well plates has become a standard practice to enable a throughput that is high enough to make sample analysis a practical process.

After the screening and selection process has resulted in a single clinical lead candidate, screening experiments are focused on exploring and determining the factors that provide maximum stability for this candidate under relevant and stability indicating storage conditions, as well as conditions that assess or potentially predict stability during manufacture and drug delivery (e.g., route of administration, combination product configurations, devices). At this stage the purpose of formulation screening is the identification of a robustness formulation design space. It means that the stability profile of a formulation has to be examined outside the product specification (i.e., pH, protein, excipient, and surfactant concentration) and recommended storage condition, and need to include evaluation of handling conditions that are required for product hold times, sample handling during labeling and packaging, and transportation. External factors that include container surfaces of vials or syringes, an extended temperature range, as well as shear stress induced from syringe plungers and pumps need to be examined to demonstrate robustness of a given formulation. Many of these external factors, in particular the impact of container surfaces and mechanical stress factors from syringe pumps and needles (e.g., cavitation and shear) are difficult to simulate in multi-well plate-based high-throughput experiments. However, even though some of the stress-simulating experiments are to be conducted outside a high-throughput compatible setup, the aggregation and organization of the test samples and their preparation can be automated, as well as their transfer to high-throughput compatible platforms for a variety of analytical measurements. As mentioned earlier, plate-based screening allows formulation scientists to expand the number of formulation compositions, storage conditions, and characterization assays. However, it is critical for a formulation scientist to demonstrate comparability between data obtained from plate-based high-throughput experiments and data derived from more traditional screening studies that use representative drug product configurations (e.g., container type, fill volume, headspace, etc.), to demonstrate the validity of the approach and data.

Besides the expansion of a reasonable screening space and accelerated execution of experiments and analysis, the modular design of the high-throughput screening methodology introduces greater flexibility to the drug development process. Ideally, formulation scientist develop a number of different modules that can be recruited for the assessment of product specific properties by applying the appropriate automation tools for sample preparation and handling, as well as the appropriate stability indicating assay and data processing programs. In Fig. 1.3, a diagram with various possible high-throughput modules is shown at the top of the graph, indicating the number of candidates and formulations to be screened at a particular stage of drug development. There are various module types and assays that can be used to screen formulations or candidates at a specific phase of development. At the beginning of the development cycle, the number of candidates could be fairly high and it makes practical sense to screen only few formulation conditions for all candidates. The number of stress and analytical methods can be also selected to limit the characterization to only the most critical candidate attributes. The formulation development during the early phases of development, however, should be characterized by an extensive analysis of a wide variety of formulations and product quality attributes to obtain the comprehensive understanding of a molecule's stability properties. To this end, depending on molecule type and stage of development, and the information that needs to be obtained, various modules of a high-throughput system can be specifically selected and applied.

The total number of samples that is required for a formulation development study is determined by the sum of the number of formulation types and number of formulation conditions. Ideally, going downstream in the development process, the screening is being limited to the combination of one molecule and one formulation that represents the best fit for a specific dosage form and route of delivery. In reality, however, a defined space of formulation conditions needs to be evaluated and to satisfy stability robustness requirements. Data obtained by multidimensional high-throughput characterization studies can define such a formulation space with statistically justified confidence intervals and robustness limits. The conclusions can be made not only about the operational space but also about the space where stability goes beyond acceptable parameters.

Furthermore, it is essential to store and manage the data that are generated by a high-throughput process in a database or other appropriate data and information management systems (e.g., electronic laboratory notebook, data warehouse, etc.). The advantage is that if data are stored in a database, they can be used not only in a manual

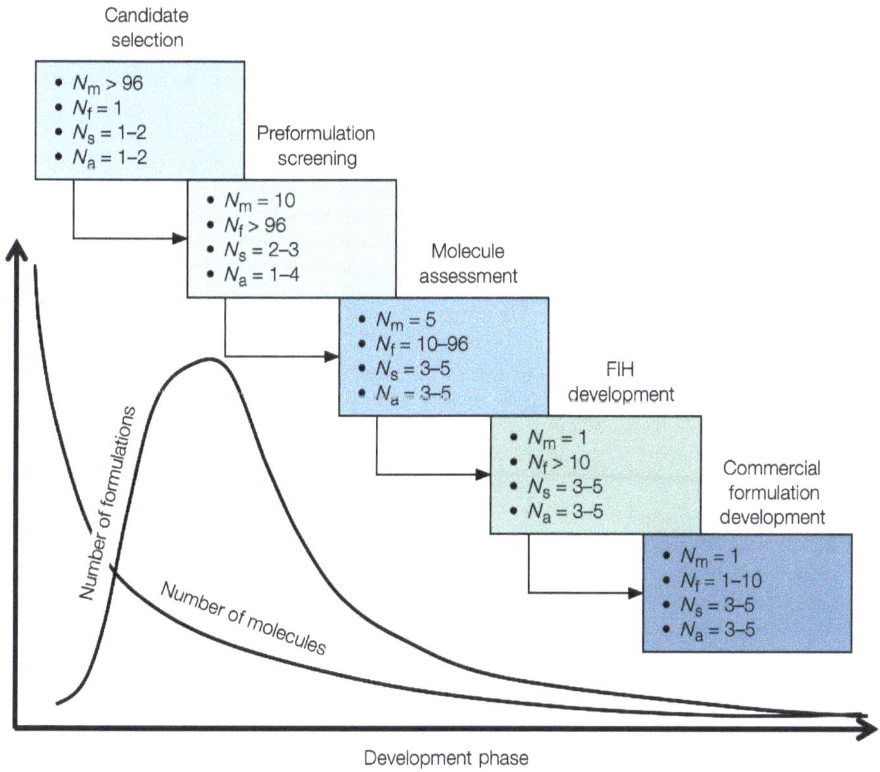

Figure 1.3 Modular structure of high-throughput analytical and characterization tools with flexibility for applications in different phases of development. N_m, number of molecules; N_f, number of formulations; N_s, number of stress methods; N_a, number of analytical methods.

and empirical process but also in a more targeted and selective manner to facilitate more in-depth analyses of a molecule or more comprehensively across molecules within a class of molecules (modality). These increasingly growing "historical" data sets can then be leveraged by stability acceptance criteria to inform the formulation scientist about a molecule's stability profile.

Last but not least, efficiencies in formulation development can be further increased if high-throughput processes are paired with formulation platform development approaches. The advantage of a platform process is that the formulation space and its components, as well as the set of analytical techniques and assays are standardized and consistent throughout formulation development. Since a platform formulation process is nonproduct specific but agnostic to a class of molecules, a high-throughput process is not limited by a "one molecule at a time" approach but can accommodate multiple molecules in a high-throughput batch workflow, executing the entire process for multiple molecules from sample preparation and handling all the way through analysis and data processing in an automated, fast, and highly efficient process. This gain in efficiency is not limited to early phase development. If "end-to-end" platform approaches are in place, directly targeting commercialization at the beginning of development, a well designed high-throughput process is not only increasing efficiency but creates greater alignment between early and late stage development activities and requirements.

References

[1] A.S. Rathore, Roadmap for implementation of quality by design (QbD) for biotechnology products, Trends Biotechnol. 27 (9) (2009) 546–553.

[2] B. Horvath, M. Mun, M.W. Laird, Characterization of a monoclonal antibody cell culture production process using a quality by design approach, Mol. Biotechnol. 45 (3) (2010) 203–206.

[3] K. Ng, N. Rajagopalan, Application of quality by design and risk assessment principles for the development of formulation design space, in: A.S. Rathore, R. Mhatre (Eds.), Quality by Design for Biopharmaceuticals: Principles and Case Studies, John Wiley & Sons, Inc., Hoboken, NJ, USA. http://dx.doi.org/10.1002/9780470466315. Chapter 9.

[4] H.M.L. Larsen, H. Trnka, H. Grohganz, Formation of mannitol hemihydrate in freeze-dried protein formulations—A design of experiment approach, Int. J. Pharm. 460 (1) (2014) 45–52.

[5] <http://www.tecan.com/page/content/index.asp?MenuID=2108&ID=3366&Menu=1&Item=21.1.9>.

[6] <http://www.freeslate.com/applications/life-science/large-molecule>.

[7] S. Kreusch, S. Schwedler, B. Tautkus, G.A. Cumme, A. Horn, UV measurements in microplates suitable for high-throughput protein determination, Anal. Biochem. 313 (2) (2003) 208–215.

[8] K.A. Chan, S.G. Kazarian, Fourier transform infrared imaging for high-throughput analysis of pharmaceutical formulations, J. Comb. Chem. 7 (2) (2005) 185–189.

[9] V. Plotnikov, A. Rochalski, M. Brandts, J.F. Brandts, S. Williston, V. Frasca, et al., An autosampling differential scanning calorimeter instrument for studying molecular interactions, Assay Drug Dev. Technol. 1 (1) (2002) 83–90.

[10] E. Chapman, C.H. Wong, A pH sensitive colorimetric assay for the high-throughput screening of enzyme inhibitors and substrates: a case study using kinases, Bioorg. Med. Chem. 10 (3) (2002) 551–555.

[11] S.A. Sundberg, High-throughput and ultra-high-throughput screening: solution-and cell-based approaches, Curr. Opin. Biotechnol. 11 (1) (2000) 47–53.

[12] C.D. Bevan, R.S. Lloyd, A high-throughput screening method for the determination of aqueous drug solubility using laser nephelometry in microtiter plates, Anal. Chem. 72 (8) (2000) 1781–1787.

[13] Y. He, E.S. Yeung, High-throughput screening of kinase inhibitors by multiplex capillary electrophoresis with UV absorption detection, Electrophoresis 24 (1–2) (2003) 101–108.

[14] M.A. Capelle, R. Gurny, T. Arvinte, High throughput screening of protein formulation stability: practical considerations, Eur. J. Pharm. Biopharm. 65 (2) (2007) 131–148.

[15] H. Zhao, O. Graf, N. Milovic, X. Luan, M. Bluemel, M. Smolny, et al., Formulation development of antibodies using robotic system and high-throughput laboratory (HTL), J. Pharm. Sci. 99 (5) (2010) 2279–2294.

[16] S. Basavaraj, G.V. Betageri, Can formulation and drug delivery reduce attrition during drug discovery and development—review of feasibility, benefits and challenges, Acta Pharm. Sinic. B 4 (1) (2014) 3–17.

Early candidate selection and formulation development

2

2.1 Screening for colloidal and conformational stability

The final candidate selection is a very important research milestone indicating the completion of lead-candidate selection and the beginning of the preclinical, first-in-human development phase for a new drug. During this phase of development, the decision to advance the lead candidate molecule into the clinic should be based on a comprehensive data package comprising data from a cross-functional team of experts from a variety of disciplines, such as discovery research, drug substance and drug product development, as well as toxicology, manufacturing, regulatory, and clinical functions. A decision to advance a candidate molecule is never based on a single set of results, but rather is made on a set of development data that demonstrate product manufacturability, stability, safety, and efficacy. Formulation selection also plays a critical part in early development and should be performed with the same thoroughness as the selection of drug candidates.

The process of early drug candidate selection has been heavily dependent on biological activity. Bioactivity screening methods are generally based on cell or cell-free systems, which to a large extent are amenable to automation and high-throughput workflows. The identification of a lead candidate is followed by toxicology, pharmacokinetics, and drug metabolism studies to predict drug dosing, safety, and efficacy. These often costly and time-consuming studies used to be mostly low throughput and required milliliters of solution volume. Nowadays they are performed in multi-well plates with 384, 1024, and more wells, using only micro and even nanoliters of reagents. The miniaturization enables screening of hundreds or thousands of compounds per day. Many liquid-dispensing systems and detection systems are compatible with microtiter plate-reader formats, and advances in robotics and integral chip-based technologies have made it possible to develop and automate many types of high-throughput methodologies. Many methods for both sample handling and detection, originally designed for small molecules, have also found applications in biopharmaceutical development. Some properties of small molecule formulations are similar to biopharmaceutical formulations. For example, solubility and aggregation propensity are critical attributes for both protein and small molecule formulations, and those factors require thoughtful and thorough assessments during early screening of candidates and development of suitable formulations. However, the solubility and aggregation propensity of proteins are generally less predictable than for small molecules.

Early candidate development, in its majority, is still lacking methodologies for the thorough analysis and development of formulation properties that provide appropriate stability for drug substance and drug product storage, handling, and transportation.

High-Throughput Formulation Development of Biopharmaceuticals. DOI: http://dx.doi.org/10.1016/B978-1-907568-63-3.00002-5

Poor solubility can produce errors and artifacts by interfering with the measurement of various parameters, such as protein concentration or binding activity, which in turn may cause misinterpretations of assay results. Due to overlapping, ultraviolet (UV) absorbance bands that originate from the absorbance of protein in solution at 280 nm and wavelength-dependent (Raleigh-scatter) absorption of aggregated protein between 280 and 360 nm that is typical of particulate matter, protein precipitation can result in an overestimation of the protein concentration although the actual protein amount in solution is reduced. Furthermore, the formation of soluble aggregates can significantly increase or decrease bioactivity and induce immunogenicity [1–3]. Understanding the dependence of solubility on pH and ionic strength can facilitate improved expression and protein recovery. Due to the complex nature of proteins it is not straightforward to develop a formulation that not only provides optimal solubility for a specific protein but also is universally applicable to a class of molecules. For example, monoclonal antibodies (mAbs), as a molecule class, are very similar in structure but are characterized by physical attributes that result in stability and solubility properties that are quite different from each other. In some cases just a few point mutations can dramatically change an antibody's solubility [4]. Very early toxicological studies on animals require protein candidates to be monomeric and soluble in order to evaluate their activity and toxicity as accurately as possible. Similarly, pharmacokinetics and pharmacodynamics studies demand soluble and stable formulations to produce meaningful data.

Protein solubility can be characterized as thermodynamically and kinetically driven. Both types play a critical role in downstream processes that involve inclusion body refolding, hydrophobic interaction chromatography, and formulation development. High-throughput screening methods and automated liquid-handling systems have been successfully used to rapidly evaluate the apparent solubility of lysozyme to find the formulation components and formulation composition that delivered maximal protein solubility [5]. The studied variables were pH, ionic strength, and excipient concentration. Parameter interactions were determined between pH and temperature. The key result of this work revealed that the temperature effect was stronger than the effect of pH and that increasing the ionic strength of the formulation induced changes in the apparent solubility for all systems. PEG 300 and Tween 20 increased the apparent solubility of lysozyme at high salt concentrations. Maximal apparent solubility was achieved in the presence of excipients such as sorbitol and sucrose.

The screening for solubility and the propensity of aggregation is one of the main priorities for the candidate selection process, the first steps of protein purification, and sample preparation for other methods. During the early development phases of lead-candidate selection, the number of candidates is large and the amount of proteins available is small. Therefore, the methods applied should be able to accommodate small sample volumes and should be able to reliably process large sample sizes in a relatively short period of time. It is an interesting phenomenon that old biochemical methods that have been out of vogue for some time have been rediscovered to evaluate colloidal stability and solubility of biopharmaceutical products. One method to assess colloidal stability of proteins in solution is to test their propensity to precipitate. Precipitation can be induced by addition of salts or other chemicals, which is a methodology that has been used in protein purification for several decades. For example, ammonium sulfate is a commonly used agent to induce precipitation of proteins [6]. However, precipitation by ammonium sulfate is dependent on a number of formulation factors. One disadvantage of using ammonium sulfate is its pH dependency. The optimal pH for precipitating proteins with ammonium sulfate is around 5.2. This prevents its usage for formulations with an optimal pH far from pH 5.2 or which are not stable at pH 5.2. Ammonium sulfate acts as a salting-out agent and to be effective it requires relatively high salt concentrations. Another precipitation agent, which has been used in solubility screening studies as an alternative to ammonium sulfate, is polyethylene glycol (PEG). The mechanism of PEG-induced precipitation is different from that of the ammonium sulfate-induced mechanism. PEG acts by the mechanism of the excluded volume model, in which water molecules are excluded from the interface between interacting proteins, which in turn causes proteins to aggregate and subsequently precipitate [7]. This methodology has been successfully applied to screen for solubility of therapeutic antibodies in a number of applications [8]. In liquid–liquid phase separation experiments, PEG can be used as a precipitation agent to estimate protein solubility as a function of PEG concentration by its effect on the liquid–liquid phase boundary of the binary protein–water system [9]. In other experiments, PEG can be used to determine a protein's native state solubility as a function of excipient type under long-term storage conditions (i.e., 2–8°C) [10]. The advantage of using precipitation agents like PEG is that screening for protein solubility can be conducted in different formulation compositions and storage conditions, in multiple solutions without applying any stresses such as agitation or elevated temperature. Applying these types of external stress conditions leads to structural perturbations and protein unfolding, which are better suited to determine the conformational stability of proteins and need to be avoided for experiments designed to test colloidal stability under relevant long-term storage conditions, which require the assessment of native state protein–protein interactions.

The methodology of rapid high-throughput screening can be used as an experimental tool to determine protein solubility profiles for the comparison of protein formulations and ranking of formulation components and properties; e.g., buffer types and pH. It is therefore a good fit for automated study and analysis platforms for formulation screening experiments [11]. These types of precipitation methods can be easily incorporated into high-throughput processes by utilizing multi-well plate formats. The level of precipitation can be characterized by measuring the remaining protein concentration in the soluble phase after separation from the precipitated phase by centrifugation. Many types of commercially available plate readers can perform absorbance measurements at a wavelength of 280 nm. The linearity of the absorbance measurement follows the Beer–Lambert law, which means that the absorbance signal, depending on the extinction coefficient of a particular protein, may not be higher than approximately 1–2 absorbance units. For formulations of highly concentrated proteins the concentration measurements have to be performed in cuvettes or in solutions with very short optical path lengths. Alternatively, high-throughput size-exclusion high-performance liquid chromatography (SE-HPLC) systems can be used to determine protein concentrations of highly concentrated formulations. The relatively high hydrophobicity of PEG molecules can be a problem for the execution of certain analytical methods. As mentioned above, to be effective, precipitation agents like ammonium sulfate and PEG need to be used at relatively high concentrations. Therefore, extra caution should be taken to make sure that these precipitating agents do not interfere with the protein's interaction with the column resin, which could negatively impact the quality and validity of the chromatographic profile. Usually, the ammonium sulfate concentration required to precipitate proteins is not dependent on the protein concentration. In cases where protein precipitation is dependent on protein concentration other factors impacting stability may be responsible for reduced protein stability or lack of protein solubility.

Applications for the assessment of conformational stability of proteins recruit conditions that induce structural perturbations or protein unfolding. The conformational stability of proteins is important to be understood to make sure that the production and purification processes are compatible with a protein's stability limits. Although the majority of therapeutic proteins are produced in mammalian cells, proteins are also produced in bacteria. Protein production in bacteria, utilizing rapid fermentation processes, results in large quantities of recombinant protein being deposited in insoluble inclusion bodies. The solubilization of these aggregated protein inclusion bodies causes denaturation and often leads to low amounts of correctly refolded native protein. Therefore, the production yields of active protein product are limited by the formation of inactive misfolded species, as well as aggregates [12].

One of the most obvious and easy-to-apply stresses to challenge conformational stability is temperature. The determination of a protein's thermal stability is a useful parameter in the selection of therapeutic candidates, produced in both bacteria and mammalian cells. Proteins with greater stability at elevated temperatures have a better chance to maintain structural integrity and survive the different stresses that are introduced or induced by the production, purification, and fill-finish process. Conformational stability may influence the ratio of folded and unfolded protein in a cell during production and the expression levels and overall titer. Inherently, unfolded or partially unfolded proteins have a higher tendency to aggregate because of the interaction of exposed hydrophobic surface areas and residues, which tend to strongly interact and collapse onto each other in aqueous solutions. Unfolding or conformational changes can be induced by a variety of factors such as temperature, pH, surface interactions, impurities, and the presence of denaturing agents. These factors can have an additive or even synergistic effect on protein unfolding. During the purification process, surface interactions provide one of the sources for conformational changes; e.g., filters [13], chromatographic resins, fill lines, and storage containers like glass and plastic vials and syringes. Formulation components, especially surfactants, can change protein–surface interactions [14]. Both native and non-native mechanisms can be involved to promote protein interactions with surfaces, but the most common and typically irreversible protein–surface interaction mechanisms include conformational changes.

One of the main methods for measuring the unfolding temperature of proteins is differential scanning calorimetry (DSC). DSC is a relatively low-throughput method and it requires >0.1 mg of protein per experiment. Various modifications of the original

DSC instrument design have made it possible to run experiments with smaller sample volumes and with the help of autosamplers in an automated format. Automation options are available on such instruments as the VP-Capillary DSC Platform from MicroCal (Worcestershire, UK), the PerkinElmer (Waltham, Massachusetts) PYRIS Diamond DSC Autosampler, or the TA Instruments (New Castle, Delaware) Nano DSC Autosampler System. The addition of autosamplers has significantly decreased the need for manual sample preparation and execution of experiments. In some cases automated data analysis tools are also included to obtain and process acquired data more seamlessly and faster. Advances in miniaturization and microfluidic technology created the basis for array-based, higher throughput calorimetry on microchips [15,16] or microplates [17]. Microtechnologies are not commercialized yet and many laboratory prototypes are under development and in various test phases. They are all aiming at low sample volumes and high sensitivity detection. Microelectromechanical systems (MEMS) can perform measurements with volumes as little as 2 µL of protein solution. The sensitivity of one of these DSC systems has reached 5 mg/mL and continues to improve [18].

In recent years several new high-throughput assays have been developed to screen the thermostability of proteins. An interesting method has been applied by Ghaemmaghami et al. to screen protein stability of unpurified proteins with hydrogen/deuterium (H/D) exchange mass spectrometry [19] in a rapid, high-throughput fashion. In this method, cell lysates are exposed to different concentrations of the denaturant guanidine hydrochloride and the induced amount of protein unfolding is determined by measuring the rate of H/D exchange with matrix-assisted laser desorption/ionization (MALDI) mass spectrometry. It was shown that the determined free energy of folding (ΔG_f) agreed well with the ΔG_f values obtained with more conventional measurements using circular dichroism (CD) spectroscopy. This method is also applicable to determine the effect of pH, excipients, and other stabilizers on the free energy of folding of purified proteins. In formulation development it is important to understand what factors destabilize and what factors stabilize the structural integrity of a protein or peptide. Although the advantage of CD measurements is that its signal is directly related to the protein structure, it is a measurement that is not high throughput. The use of plates is not practical because CD measurements require cuvettes with high-quality optics and very short path lengths for the determination of a protein's secondary structure, which are not available in a plate-based setup. But similar to the modern DSC setup it is possible to automate the process of sample handling and optical measurement to significantly increase the throughput. It has been demonstrated that the accuracy and precision of a CD spectrometer that is equipped with a robotic liquid-handling system and an optical flow-through cell is comparable with the data quality of low-throughput instruments [20]. An automated CD spectrometer like this allows unattended measurements of 384 samples and is therefore applicable for large-scale formulation screening studies. Both far- and near-ultraviolet CD measurements, depending on the path length of the cuvette chosen, require sample volumes between 100 and 1000 µL, respectively. The instrument uses plate holders and a cell cartridge that houses a low-birefringence fused silica flow-through cell with a discrete optical path length of 0.2, 0.5, or 10 mm. The plates are maintained at particular temperatures with the help of Peltier units and aluminum blocks designed to provide reliable temperature control for 2 mL deep-well plates. The temperature of the flow cell is controlled separately.

Differential scanning fluorimetry (DSF) is another technique to assess the conformational stability of proteins by utilizing extrinsic fluorescence probes. Pantoliano et al. [21] measured the change of extrinsic fluorescence in the presence of a small-molecule ligand to measure ligand-induced protein stabilization [21]. Ligand binding to a protein induces a thermal shift or a shift of the unfolding temperature to higher temperatures, which is indicative of a protein with greater conformational stability. In addition, thermodynamics have been used to calculate binding constants and to rank ligand-binding affinities. This technique has been also applied in a high-throughput format to evaluate multiphasic-unfolding behavior resulting from subsaturating binding of ligands [22]. Multiphasic unfolding, detected by this method, is a strong indication of a heterogeneous protein solution, which often interferes with a protein's ability to crystalize. Therefore, extrinsic fluorescent probe measurements have utility in screening solution compositions optimal for protein crystallization. To this end, the change in fluorescence intensity of an extrinsic probe is measured during a temperature scan and the midpoint of the intensity transition determines the melting temperature (T_m) or the temperature of hydrophobic exposure (T_h) of the hydrophobic residues or areas of the unfolding protein the fluorescent probe is interacting with. Fig. 2.1 shows a number of typical DSF scans that were obtained to screen the thermostability of different mAb formulations. In this particular study, a 96-well plate format was used to screen different formulations of a single mAb molecule [23]. The fluorescent probe used for this study was SYPRO Orange. The final protein concentration was 1 mg/mL after dilution. SYPRO Orange was diluted 1:5000 in the protein solution. The temperature screen was performed on a BioRad CFX96 thermal cycler (Bio-Rad Laboratories, Inc., Hercules, California). The fluorescence was measured while the temperature was increased from 20°C to 95°C in 0.2°C increments. Samples were exposed to each temperature for 3 seconds before measuring the fluorescence signal. The temperature of hydrophobic exposure (T_h) was determined from the peak(s) of the first derivatives of the fluorescence transition curves that were calculated using the Bio-Rad *CFX Manager* software (Bio-Rad Laboratories, Inc., Hercules, California). In another study [24], a comparison with thermostability measurements using DSC revealed a good correlation between the T_h and the melting temperature T_m. For comparison the DSC and DSF signals versus temperature plots for different buffers and pH values are shown in Fig. 2.2. According to these unfolding transitions it seems that the onset of DSF signal is occurring slightly before the onset of the DSC signal. Particularly at higher pH values (>pH 7.0) the DSF transitions occur at lower temperatures than the DSC transitions. Nonetheless, as illustrated in Fig. 2.3, the T_h versus T_m plot generated for various formulations shows a fairly good correlation between the two techniques. The DSF data discussed here were derived from a screening study comprised of four mAbs formulated in 84 formulations each. The protein concentration in each of the wells of the 96-well plate was 0.1 mg/mL. To determine the sensitivity of the DSF method, a solution of a fully denatured antibody was used to monitor the fluorescence signal of an antibody with fully exposed hydrophobic residues,

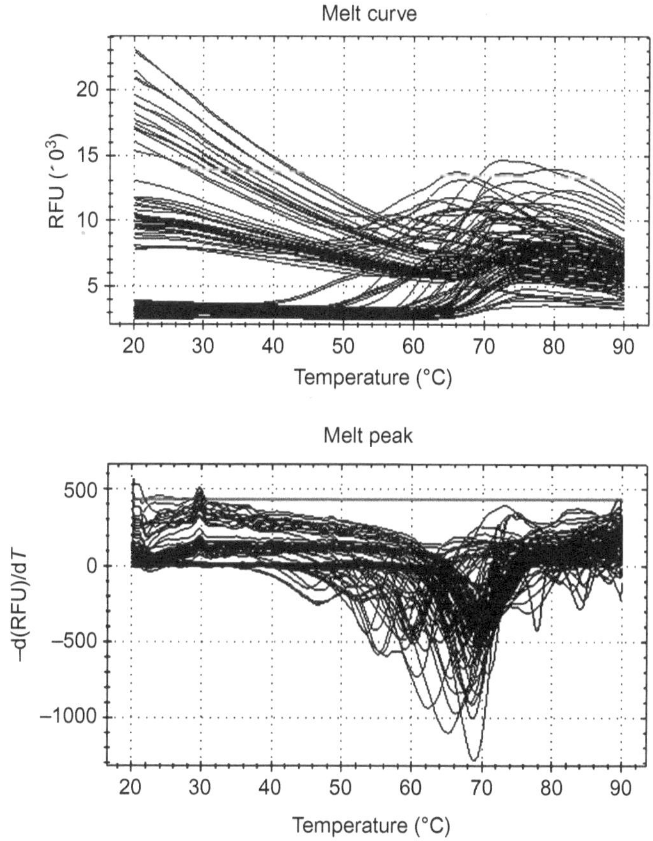

Figure 2.1 Fluorescence of SYPRO Orange is shown as a function of temperature (top panel) for 96 different formulations. The bottom panel shows the first derivative of fluorescence versus temperature data presented in the top panel. The values at the transition minima at the lowest temperatures were used to determine the temperature of hydrophobic exposure T_h.

allowing full access for the hydrophobic fluorescent probe to interact. The observed change in fluorescence signal correlated well with the level of hydrophobic exposure. It is noteworthy to mention that in the mAb formulations presented here, the SYPRO Orange fluorescent probe produced a relatively low fluorescence background under native conditions, specifically in the IgG1 and IgG2 formulations. Consequently, the first transition at the lowest temperature is the most visible in DSF scans. For other types of proteins and formulations the fluorescence background of the fluorescent probe may be different and appropriate control experiments need to be performed to understand the sensitivity and dynamic range of the DSF signal. The results of the study indicated a pH effect on the T_h values for different mAb molecules. The other objective of this study was to compare and differentiate the conformational stability of the four mAbs in the 84 formulations as a function of various formulation

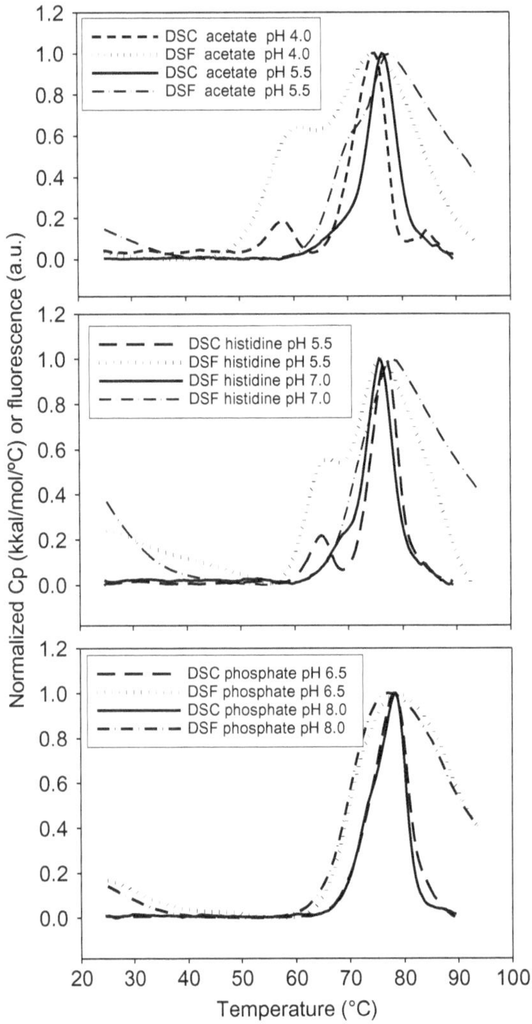

Figure 2.2 Comparison of DSC and DSF signals as a function of temperature for different buffers and pH values. The low temperature transition corresponds to the unfolding of the C_H2 domain.

Source: From F. He, S. Hogan, R.F. Latypov, L.O. Narhi, V.I. Razinkov, High throughput thermostability screening of monoclonal antibody formulations, J. Pharm. Sci. 99 (4) (2010) 1707–1720, Figure 3.

factors. According to Fig. 2.4, the unfolding temperature of the antibody formulations increased with increasing pH until the pH values reached ~6.5. At pH values above 6.5, the unfolding temperature became pH independent. One explanation may be that above pH 6.5 the unfolding temperature of the C_H2 domain starts to overlap with the unfolding temperature of the more stable Fab domain, which is much less sensitive to pH changes than the C_H2 domain. The effect of excipients on T_h is shown in

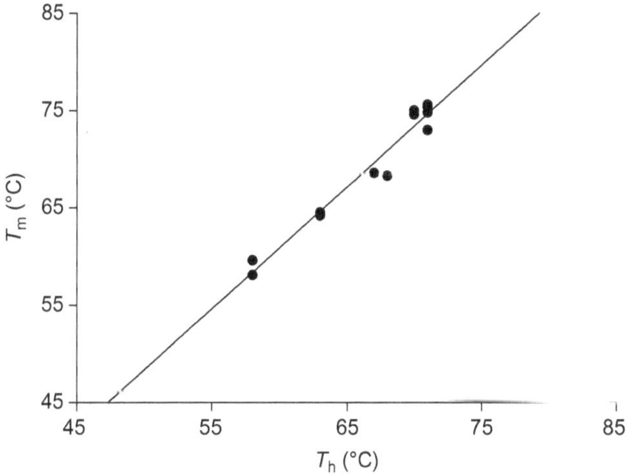

Figure 2.3 Correlation between T_h and T_m. Samples containing mAb1 or mAb2 (both at 0.5 mg/mL) were prepared in a variety of solutions including: 40 mM acetate, pH 4.0 and 5.5; 40 mM histidine, pH 5.5 and 7.0; 40 mM phosphate, pH 6.5 and 8.0. The transition midpoint of the first derivative curves, created from the DSF profiles, was used to determine the T_h values. The T_m values were determined from the transition in the DSC thermogram that occurs at the lowest temperature. Linear regression analysis yielded a linearity correlation coefficient $R^2 = 0.9605$.
Source: From F. He, S. Hogan, R.F. Latypov, L.O. Narhi, V.I. Razinkov, High throughput thermostability screening of monoclonal antibody formulations, J. Pharm. Sci. 99 (4) (2010) 1707–1720, Figure 4.

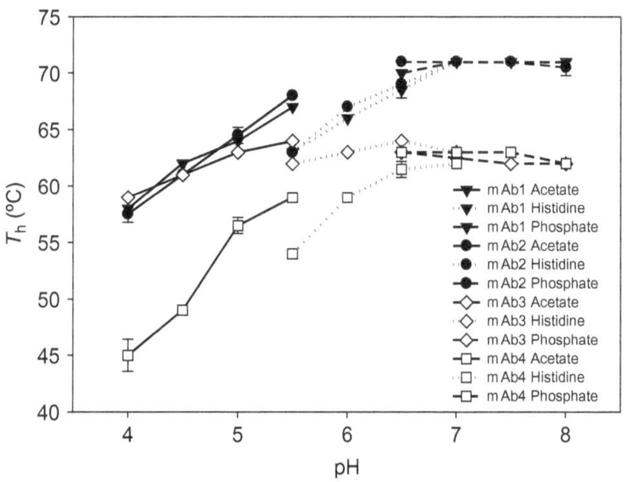

Figure 2.4 Shown are the T_h values as a function of pH for different mAb molecules in various buffers.
Source: From F. He, S. Hogan, R.F. Latypov, L.O. Narhi, V.I. Razinkov, High throughput thermostability screening of monoclonal antibody formulations, J. Pharm. Sci. 99 (4) (2010) 1707–1720, Figure 5.

Fig. 2.5, indicating that different excipients and excipient types have very different effects on the unfolding temperature of the four antibodies in this study. The presence of salt reduces protein stability, particularly at low pH. The general trend is that salt has a destabilizing effect; sucrose and sorbitol have a stabilizing positive effect; proline and glycine have only a small effect on protein stability. The effect of arginine on protein stability was pH and protein dependent. Arginine only had a small negative effect on protein stability for one of the mAbs (mAb1) and only at pH 4.0 (Fig. 2.5A). For the formulations of the other antibodies (mAb2, mAb3, and mAb4) the effect of arginine was increasingly destabilizing with decreasing pH values (Fig. 2.5B–D). This study also revealed that the IgG1 antibodies seem to be more stable than other IgG antibody subclasses. In summary, high-throughput screening of various mAb molecules and formulations resulted in a pool of conformational stability data that enabled the differentiation between different antibodies and formulation components, as well as molecule selection and formulation optimization.

Typically, T_h values are determined for the least stable protein domain; i.e., the domain with the lowest melting temperature of a multidomain protein. It is difficult to resolve the T_h transitions for any of the other more stable domains, because the fluorescence signal emitted by the fluorescent probe interacting with the unfolded domain overlaps with the signals from interactions with other, more stable, domains. Quenching at elevated temperatures also contributes to overall loss in fluorescence signal. The presence of detergent in formulations may also interfere with SYPRO Orange and some other extrinsic fluorescent probes. However, new probes, insensitive to surfactants have been introduced to avoid this problem [25]. Surfactants are widely used in mAb formulations as a stabilizer. But fluorescence of traditionally used probes such as SYPRO Orange is significantly increased in the presence of micelles formed by surfactants, concealing the signal of protein unfolding. The new molecular probe 4-(dicyanovinyl)julolidine (DCVJ) has been employed in a study of antibody formulations containing polysorbate 20, polysorbate 80, or poloxamer 188. The DCVJ-based method was able to determine the melting temperature of antibodies in formulations where SYPRO Orange failed. The use of control formulations without protein is critical for the accurate determination of the unfolding temperature, specifically for measuring the onset of the fluorescence signal at the temperature when it increases above the fluorescence background. Using DCVJ for DSF measurements expands the number and variety of surfactant-containing formulations that can be screened for optimal stability. A good review on high-throughput stability screening methods has been published by Thomas J. Magliery [26]. One of the methods mentioned in the review is based on quantitative cysteine reactivity, which has been developed to explore the conformational changes of proteins and to measure the free energy of folding (ΔG_f). The method uses thiol-reactive probes to modify cysteine residues that are initially buried inside folded proteins. The structurally protected cysteine residues can be exposed to the solution and labeled by the external probes by temperature-induced partial or complete unfolding. The difference in free energy between the folded and unfolded state is determined by the amount of cysteine modification as a function of temperature. The benefit of using the cysteine reactivity assay for protein stability measurements is that it only requires picomoles of protein sample.

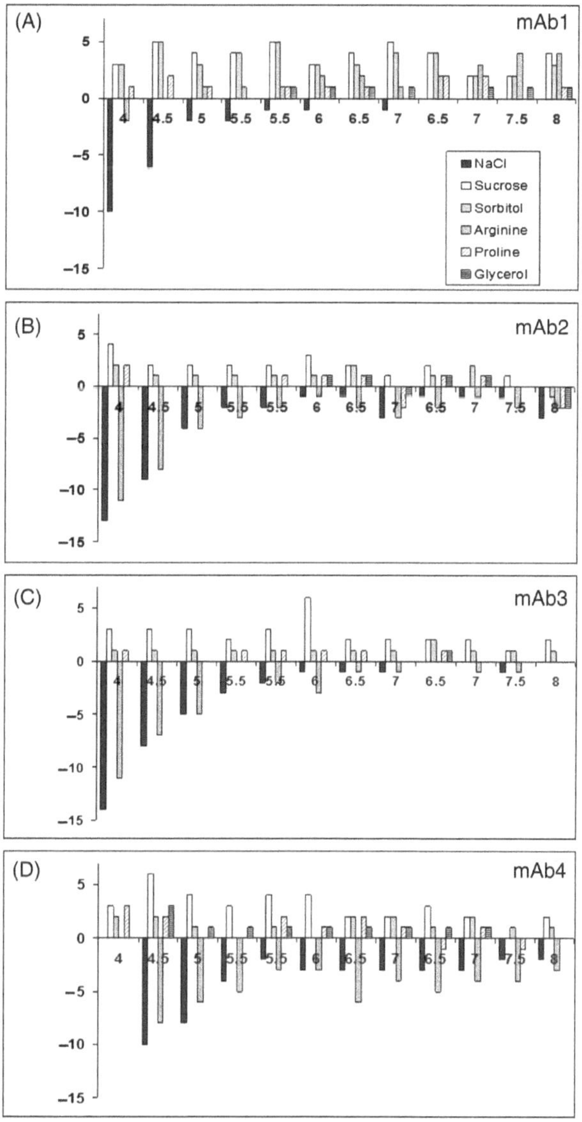

Figure 2.5 Shown is the effect of excipients and pH on the change in temperature of hydrophobic exposure (ΔT_h) for four different mAb molecules (A–D). DSF measurements were performed with these four mAbs in overall 84 different formulations at a protein concentration of 0.1 mg/mL. ΔT_h was determined by subtracting the T_h values obtained in excipient free buffers from excipient containing buffers.
Source: From F. He, S. Hogan, R.F. Latypov, L.O. Narhi, V.I. Razinkov, High throughput thermostability screening of monoclonal antibody formulations, J. Pharm. Sci. 99 (4) (2010) 1707–1720, Figure 6.

Multiple formulation samples can be gradually heated and simultaneously analyzed by a light scattering detector (e.g., OPTIM 2 light scattering detector manufactured by Avacta Analytical (Wetherby, UK)). The instrument screens small volumes of samples simultaneously for determining both a protein's unfolding and aggregation temperature.

The use of fluorescent probes to detect protein aggregation and to aid formulation development is utilized in the ProteoStat protein aggregation assay, which is based on the Synergy Mx multimode microplate reader (BioTek Instruments, Inc., Winooski, Vermont). The ProteoStat assay provides a simple methodology to detect protein aggregation. Samples are analyzed on multi-well microplates using conventional protein aggregation detection dyes such as Thioflavin T, as well as the ProteoStat detection reagent. According to the manufacturer, the detection limit of aggregated protein is less than 1%. Different types of protein aggregates can be detected and quantified in formulations with different pH values and buffer compositions within a dynamic range of two orders of magnitude. Alternatively, the level of protein aggregation in a small volume format can be assessed with new electrophoresis methods. Advancements in material sciences have enabled the recent development of new silica colloidal crystals, which were specifically designed to decrease the time to separate protein aggregates during electrophoresis [27]. Compared to traditional polyacrylamide gels (PAGs), the silica colloidal crystals operate at higher numbers of theoretical plates and migration velocities. Although the selectivity of a PAG is higher, the band broadening in colloidal crystals is much smaller. Plate heights of 0.15 μm for monomeric antibodies and 0.42 μm for antibody dimers are typical for this type of material. The time for separating monomer from dimer on colloidal crystal media is five times shorter than the total run time required for the same separation by size-exclusion high-performance liquid chromatography and is accomplished over a distance of only 6.5 mm. This makes colloidal crystal-based electrophoresis a well-suited high-throughput method for the fast assessment of protein aggregation at a miniaturized scale.

Another way to evaluate protein formulation stability is to test its resistance to denaturation by chemical agents in order to predict aggregation propensity. The method of chemical denaturation has significant advantages in comparison with thermal denaturation methods like DSC, where irreversible aggregation at high temperatures prevents the calculation of thermodynamic parameters necessary for accurate evaluation of conformational stability. Protein denaturation can be measured with the help of intrinsic fluorescence or circular dichroism (CD) in a high-throughput format. In general, the results determined by chemical denaturation correlate well with the propensity to aggregate under aggregation-accelerating conditions, and, therefore, can be used for the screening of multiple antibody formulations [28].

The formation of large proteinaceous particles is difficult to monitor and quantify. Conventional size-based chromatography is not applicable for the measurement of protein aggregates in the micrometer size range. The techniques such as asymmetrical field-flow fractionation or analytical ultracentrifugation are not suited for high-throughput analysis. Other methods can be automated but still require relatively high amounts of protein for reliable analysis. One method that can be automated and operated at relatively high throughput to characterize and count protein particles is label-free flow cytometry [29]. This method has been successfully applied to the analysis of subvisible antibody particles in various formulations. Different stress conditions were used to generate particles and the results obtained by cytometry were compared with light obscuration and microflow imaging methods. In addition to the proportional correlation of total particle count with these other assays, flow cytometry allows the analysis of particles down to 500nm and can provide additional structural information. Even with a high level of automation, the majority of traditional methods for particle counting and analysis use relatively large volumes of protein sample, which may not be available at the early stages of development. Advanced techniques for particle characterization applied to the late stages will be discussed in the next chapters.

In many cases, when the number of candidates to be screened is large and the amount of protein sample is small, the selection of acceptable protein molecules can be simply limited to the elimination of the most unstable candidates. To differentiate between the candidates' stability, different types of stress can be applied sequentially to determine the precipitation propensity by measuring the amount of soluble protein left in a tested formulation. Mechanical agitation and elevated temperature are typical precipitation-inducing stresses that are applied to differentiate between protein candidates. To increase the throughput of screening, the candidates can be analyzed in the same formulation, as a mixture, by analytical assays such as cation-exchange high-performance liquid chromatography, if the charge properties of those candidates are different enough for charge-based separation [30]. Generally, the interaction between the antibodies in the mixture is minimal or nonexistent and the inherent stability of the individual antibodies can be determined. However, appropriate control experiments should be conducted to avoid aggregation as a result of protein–protein interactions between different antibodies.

2.2 Screening for viscosity

One of the significant problems complicating downstream development of biologics is high viscosity of highly concentrated protein formulations. Especially the viscosity of antibody formulations with antibody concentrations exceeding 100mg/mL creates challenges for downstream processes. Antibodies and antibody-based molecules became common biopharmaceutical products to fight diseases in different therapeutic areas such as oncology, inflammation, and others [31–33]. In general, delivery of these products requires intravenous or subcutaneous (SC) injection of large amounts of protein in relatively small-volume drug product containers. Antibody treatments include administration of large doses of protein in the range of several milligrams per kilogram of bodyweight. Considering volume restrictions of less than 1.5mL per SC injection, the concentration of protein in formulations required for sufficient efficacy is commonly reaching 100–150mg/mL. High antibody concentrations are the main reason for high viscosity, which creates various problems during downstream process development, including purification, fill-finish, storage, and delivery. It is hard to predict high viscosity of proteins based on structural information. Even small changes in sequence may lead to a different charge distribution and can result in dramatic changes in the viscosity of antibodies [34]. Other factors, like weak forces based on long-range dipole–dipole or other types of charge-based interactions, are thought to be responsible for high viscosity of protein solutions [35]. Specifically, the dependence of dipole moments on pH and protein concentration is a strong indication of dipole–dipole interactions and high viscosity of antibody formulations [36]. High viscosity in protein formulations can be reduced by changing the ionic strength or adding excipients [37,38] to disrupt charge–charge interactions. Exposure to higher temperature also decreases viscosity and can be used in purification and delivery processes.

The methods for viscosity measurements of biopharmaceutical formulations are employed in many clinical and late-stage studies. During the early stage of candidate selection, the low amounts of available material make it specifically difficult to concentrate protein in a volume large enough for viscosity measurements. The common methods for viscosity measurements have been adopted from the field of polymer chemistry, or the food, cosmetic, and other industries. These methods traditionally require large volumes of liquid or colloidal suspensions and are not designed for measurements of microliters of highly concentrated protein solutions. The most commonly used and accurate assays for measuring viscosity of protein solutions include the cone and plate method [39], the falling ball method [40], and others [41,42]. Recently a potentially rapid and nondestructive method for measuring viscosity of multiple low-volume samples has been introduced [43]. In this method the Viscosizer 200 (Malvern, Malvern, UK) instrument uses a 2D UV imaging sensor to capture data in real time. This allows the employment of unique self-referencing and averaging algorithms to eliminate lamp effects, which significantly improve the signal-to-noise ratio of the measurement. It combines ultraviolet area imaging and microcapillary viscometry. Injection time errors, common to microcapillary assays, can be overcome by a dual-pass system, in which the transit time is measured with the help of ultraviolet area imaging. Protein- and peptide-specific wavelength selection enables the analysis of protein formulations containing as little as 10 μL. A comprehensive review about viscosity issues associated with concentrated therapeutic protein solutions and rheology techniques has been published by Jezek et al. [42]. The current understanding of the specific mechanisms that lead to high viscosity and approaches to control viscosity through targeted formulation design are also presented in this review. As mentioned before the traditional methods for viscosity measurements are time consuming and require significant amounts of material, making them difficult to use for high-throughput applications. New methods have been developed to miniaturize viscosity assays. Viscometer-Rheometer-On-a-Chip (VROC) technology introduced by RheoSense Inc. (San Ramon, California) is MEMS and microfluidic chip-based viscometry technology that can measure viscosity at a volume of 100 μL. Another company, Freeslate (Sunnyvale, California) incorporated a four-channel automatic viscosity measurement system into its high-throughput workstation designed for evaluating formulations of biologics. It consumes a minimum of 100 μL of sample. The viscosity of protein solutions can also be measured with the help of commercially available capillary electrophoresis, as recently described by Allmendinger et al. [44]. Allmendinger used riboflavin as a dye in protein formulations to monitor protein movement under constant pressure. The time of migration was measured and the viscosity was determined by applying Hagen–Poiseuille's law. No electrical field was required. Experiments with different capillary lots, different capillary lengths, diameters, and instruments were tested for repeatability, robustness, linearity, and reproducibility, and produced values that compared well with viscosity data obtained by cone and plate technology. The viscosity values, reliably measured by the capillary-based method, ranged from 5 to 40cP. Advantages of using capillary-based methods include short measurement times and small sample volumes, which make this technique a good fit for high-throughput applications.

The multiplexed microfluidic viscometer for simultaneous measurement of viscosity and shear rate in multiple samples has been recently introduced [45]. The technology is based on a flow comparator with an interface between simultaneous flow streams of test and reference fluids. The location of the interface is sensitive to the viscosity difference between the two fluids. The results for Newtonian and polymeric solutions obtained by the multiplexed viscometer are comparable with the data obtained by conventional rheometers. The viscometer is able to measure viscosities from about 10^{-3} to 1 Pa·s and can perform the measurements in a high-throughput format for the rapid analysis of a wide selection of complex formulation components for formulation development and quality control.

Fluorescent molecules called molecular rotors are very sensitive to solution properties and can be used for viscosity measurements of protein formulations [46]. However, at high protein concentrations, relevant to biopharmaceutical drug products, the interaction of molecular rotors with protein can interfere with the measurement and produce incorrect results. Another method for measuring viscosity of concentrated protein solutions, more amenable for small volumes, is based on the analysis of the light scattering signal from spherical polystyrene beads that are added to the protein solution [47]. According to the Stokes–Einstein equation ($D = kT/6\pi\eta r$), for any given solution, diffusant, and temperature, the diffusion coefficient of the beads depends on the solution viscosity and the bead radius. The diffusion coefficient is measured by dynamic light scattering (DLS) [48], and with the known size of the beads it is easy to calculate the viscosity of a protein solution. The method has been applied with the help of the DynaPro Platereader DLS system (Wyatt Technology, Santa Barbara, California), which consumes ~20–50 μL of solution per plate. Screening a 96-well plate usually takes about 1–2 hours depending on the instrument parameters such as the number of acquisitions per measurement and the time required for one acquisition. The process of sample preparation is simple and straightforward. Prior to viscosity measurements, 0.5 μL of concentrated polystyrene beads with a nominal radius of 150 nm and with a density of 1.05 g/cm^3 (Thermo Scientific Inc., Fremont, California) should be added to 49.5 μL of protein solution. The protein/beads mixture is transferred in 35 μL aliquots into each well of a 384-well plate. The DLS signal, originating from beads with sizes ranging between 100 and 500 nm, is well separated from the protein signal and makes it therefore easy to determine the apparent size of a protein. The ratio of the apparent bead size, determined by DLS, to the real bead size returns the viscosity of bead-containing solution. It is important to make sure that no air bubbles are present at the bottom of each well to avoid interference with the DLS measurement. Centrifugation at 2000–3000 rpm can help to remove the bubbles. The optimal size of the beads used for viscosity measurements should be determined based on expected viscosity values. Even the smallest bead size is supposed to be large enough to effectively separate the light scattering signal of the beads from that of the protein. Very large beads may be too heavy and precipitate, causing significant interferences with the DLS measurement. Additionally, the material of the beads should have an appropriate dielectric constant range to avoid any significant nonelastic interaction of light with the beads. Many light scattering methods do not tolerate any impurities of both small- and large-sized particles that can interfere with the measurements. Therefore, a high level of purification is required for accurate measurements. Despite these disadvantages, DLS-based methods are well suited for candidate screening to select and rank molecules with a potential for high viscosity because they consume only relatively small amounts of purified protein.

In addition to DLS-based methods for viscosity measurements, there are several assays that are based on the calculation of viscosity using the diffusion coefficient. The diffusion coefficient in those methods is obtained by optical tracking of single particles with the help of a microscope and imaging software [49]. The use of a capillary flow cell and autoinjector can create a high-throughput setup for fast, small volume viscosity measurements. The disadvantages of DLS-based methods include the possibility of bead–protein interactions, which may cause aggregation and subsequent precipitation of bead–protein complexes resulting in incorrect measurements. The shear rate dependence on solution structure can also be measured by DLS. The values of such measurements, however, are interrelated to the microlevel interactions with the bead surface and can be different from shear rates measured by the cone and plate method [47]. Furthermore, in some cases fluid shear can induce conformational changes of proteins [50].

2.3 Screening for chemical stability

The typical chemical degradation pathways for proteins include oxidation, deamidation, hydrolysis, isomerization, beta-elimination, disulfide exchange, and others. Many of these modifications can be predicted with different levels of probability by sequence analysis [51]. For example, the common targets for oxidation are methionine, tryptophan, and tyrosine residues. Initial screening experiments for chemical degradations include sequence analysis and the search for so-called "hot spots," particularly reactive amino acid residue side chains, where protein modifications have a high probability to occur. In addition to the primary sequence, information about the two- and three-dimensional structure is critical for determining biochemical stability [52,53]. The effect of the three-dimensional structure on the deamidation rate of asparagine residues has been shown in a study by Capasso et al. [54]. The presented data on RNase A and two peptides with sequences similar to the asparagine containing sequence of the enzyme provided clear evidence that although the deamidation mechanism is similar for all three molecules, the deamidation rate was highly dependent on the structural properties of the molecules, with the by far slowest rates measured for RNase A. The lower deamidation rate constant for the enzyme can be explained by a reduced mobility of the asparagine side chain and side chain–side chain interactions with other nearby residues. Several computational approaches exist to find "hot spots" for more common and less common chemical modifications of proteins. The predictions of chemical degradations like oxidation and deamidation are relatively straightforward and are merely based on statistical analysis of the neighboring amino acid residue occurrences without further systematic prediction based on the entire primary sequence [55]. Other modifications require more sophisticated prediction methods. The *cis/trans* isomerization of proline plays a critical role in protein folding, cell signaling, and transmembrane active transport. Accurate prediction of proline *cis/trans* isomerization in proteins has many important applications toward the understanding of protein structure and function. One of the methods to predict proline *cis/trans* isomerization in proteins is based on support vector machines, which uses the single amino acid sequence with different local window sizes, the amino acid compositions of local sequence flanking centered proline residues, the position-specific scoring matrices extracted by PSI-BLAST, and the predicted secondary structures [56]. Aspartic acid isomerization in the complementarity determining regions (CDR) of mAbs is commonly a critical quality attribute because it is leading in many cases to diminished biological activity. Dick et al. [57] investigated the correlation between isomerization and antibody affinity, and were able to confirm that an isomerized heavy chain resulted in decreased affinity with binding constants indicating a slower on-rate in conjunction with a faster off-rate. Various formulations were screened and the effect of different formulation factors was determined. It was found that the isomerization rate was dependent on pH values as well as on the net negative charge of buffer components that can act as proton acceptors. The levels of isomerization were predicted using the Arrhenius equation and proven to be correct by comparing them to real samples.

The rate of degradation under relevant storage conditions, usually at low temperature (2–8°C), is very slow. Reaction rates measured at conditions that accelerate the isomerization rates can be extrapolated with the help of the Arrhenius equation:

$$k = A\left(\frac{-E_a}{RT}\right)$$

where k is the rate constant of a chemical reaction, E_a the activation energy, and R and T are the gas constant and temperature, respectively. The activation energy is obtained by plotting ln(k) against $1/T$ and determining the slope of the resulting line. Using the activation energy, the reaction rate constant at relevant storage conditions (2–8°C) can be estimated by extrapolation. A thorough understanding of the reaction order is required to predict the reaction rate because the amount of the degradation product does not linearly increase over time unless the reaction follows zero-order kinetics. Many chemical degradation reactions follow the Arrhenius dependence on temperature. Therefore, long-term storage stability can be predicted by exposure to higher temperature for short periods of time. However, chemical stability characteristics of proteins are often complicated by additional factors such as conformational changes at higher temperatures or native self-association at lower temperatures. Changes to the protein structure can alter the exposure of reactive residues to the solution or to other residues. In such cases more refined models are required to accurately predict chemical degradation rates. For any given protein, depending on the solution properties and storage conditions, multiple degradation pathways involving different domains and residues are actively engaged. Each degradation reaction has its own rate order and activation energy. Therefore, the type and amount of degradation products can be very different depending on whether a protein is exposed to 4°C or 37°C. At low temperatures and during long-term storage many other factors can contribute to chemical modifications. Local change in pH, surface interaction, and fluctuations of the concentration of various formulation components can cause deviations from typical Arrhenius behavior.

Traditionally, after eliminating the obvious degradation "hot spots" by site-directed mutagenesis or other protein engineering techniques, protein candidates are chemically fairly stable unless "hot spot" residues had to be left unchanged because they are critical for bioactivity. For example, some modifications in the CDR regions of mAbs are deleterious to their activity. Also legal reasons can prevent any changes in a protein's sequence. In those cases conditions can be applied that accelerate degradation reactions to test formulation compositions and properties that keep chemical modifications at a minimum. Fortunately, well-established methods are available to induce and to analyze chemical modifications of proteins. Some of these methodologies have been modified to fit the multi-well plate format and to increase the overall throughput of sample preparation and analysis. Ion-exchange high-performance liquid chromatography (IEX-HPLC) and reversed-phase high-performance liquid chromatograph in conjunction with mass spectrometry (RP-HPLC/MS) methods have been the gold standard assays to identify chemical modifications to a protein's primary sequence. Many chemical modifications produce charge variants that differ from the variants of the original molecule. Recent advancements in the development of liquid-handling instrumentation and resin materials for columns allow IEX-HPLC separations to be completed in significantly shorter time than with traditionally used methods [58]. The charge distribution of a protein molecule is an important characterization parameter because it relates to both chemical and physical modifications of a protein. Certain formulation components can alter the charge distribution by impacting the structural conformation of a protein under both appropriate storage conditions and conditions that accelerate chemical modifications or physical changes or both (i.e., salts, pH, temperature, agitation). In many cases the general pattern of chromatographic or electrophoretic charge distribution profiles is enough to monitor the effect of different formulation components and properties, as well as a variety of storage conditions on protein stability. To this end, Wheeler et al. developed a high-throughput screening assay on a microfluidic chip to analyze antibody charge variants [59]. The separation is achieved by zone electrophoresis and is about 8- to 90-fold faster than standard, low-throughput methods. The assay has been applied to a commercial high-throughput microfluidic LabChip GXII platform (Caliper, a PerkinElmer Company, Alameda, California) that performs electrophoretic separation and laser-induced fluorescence detection. A similar microchip-based high-throughput method was developed by Creamer et al. to evaluate the charge distribution profile of mAbs in various formulations with small sample volumes and short screening times [60]. The method uses microchip zone electrophoresis for separation of charge variants of fluorescently labeled antibodies. The total time of separation is about 90 seconds, which again is more than 10 times faster than the time required by conventional methods. The assay has been applied to study the effect of excipients and buffer solution properties on protein stability. The method has been also applied to investigate variations in C-terminal lysine content and the extent of antibody deamidation. With the help of design of experiments (DOE) studies, it could be demonstrated that the method has great utility as a high-throughput assay for profiling the charge variants of mAbs and investigating its dependence on formulation composition and properties. One disadvantage these methods share is the necessity to label protein with a fluorescent probe. Although the label does not change the overall charge as such, it may introduce local conformational changes, which may change the electrophoretic separation profile. In another microchip capillary zone electrophoresis application, antibody charge profiling is performed in a high-throughput format using the fluorescent probe Cy5 *N*-hydroxysuccinimide ester [61]. Similar to the above-mentioned assays, the probe makes it possible to measure fluorescence with a microchip instrument, using 96-well plates for sample preparation and analysis. The analysis takes about 80 seconds per sample and is therefore completed in about 2 hours. Charge variant resolution has been shown to be enough to separate species that differ by 0.1 pI units. The data obtained by microchip-based analysis, such as specificity, linearity, precision, and limit of detection, were comparable with the results generated by conventional capillary zone electrophoresis, demonstrating its utility for high-throughput profiling of antibody formulations.

mAbs comprise two identical light and heavy chains. A single N-glycosylation site (Asn 297) is located in both identical heavy chains in the Fc domain. Some antibodies may also contain oligosaccharides in the Fab region. The oligosaccharides in the Fc region account for about 3% of the total protein mass, but they have a major effect on functions related to drug efficacy, pharmacokinetics, stability, and immunogenicity [62–64]. Some glycoforms can increase or decrease drug efficacy [65], and therefore the structural characterization of N-glycosylation of mAbs is of critical importance for drug development. The heterogeneity of the glycans and the large variation in abundance make thorough glycan characterization of antibodies a slow and laborious process [66,67]. Many of the commercial biopharmaceuticals were developed at a time when the analysis of glycoforms was not as advanced, and the quality for characterization much lower. Glycan analysis focused on three *N*-glycans known as G0F, G1F, and G2F [68,69]. High-throughput methods for glycan analysis are difficult to develop because they require both high resolution separation between different glycoforms and high accuracy of detection. In one of the recent studies, a liquid chromatography–mass spectrometry *N*-glycan library was developed based on the structure of eight mAbs [69]. A total of 70 glycans were included in the database. The separation of *N*-glycans was achieved by a porous graphitized carbon column on a chip and the samples were analyzed by electrospray ionization hybrid quadrupole time-of-flight mass spectrometry. The library helps to identify *N*-glycan structures in a high-throughput manner by allowing the analyst to compare measured retention times and accurate masses with those listed in the database. As demonstrated by this study, most *N*-glycans are structurally very similar and only their relative abundance is molecule specific.

Another fully automated method developed for high-throughput N-glycosylation profiling and sequencing is described in the work by Váradi et al. [70]. The method has good reproducibility and a rapid sample preparation process, which is compatible with robotic sample handling systems. The method is based on the use of carboxyl coated magnetic beads to eliminate centrifugation steps and to increase efficiency. The whole process only takes a couple of hours and the generated results compared well with results obtained from methods with traditional glycan sample preparation techniques.

Glycosylation of an IgG antibody's Fc domain is critical for effector functions. The glycosylation profile, representing the relative abundance of the individual *N*-glycan structures, also has an important impact on the selection of sufficiently stable formulations. Considering the various processing, handling, and storage conditions encountered during development, high-throughput methods to monitor antibody glycosylation are desired for fast optimization and profiling of drug product. The development of a fully automated high-throughput technique based on glycopeptide characterization has been recently described by Reusch et al. [71]. Antibody samples were prepared using 96-well plates. The IgG molecules were purified from fermentation broths through a Protein A capture step followed by trypsin digestion. Solid-phase extraction was used to purify the glycopeptides and the samples were analyzed by electrospray ionization mass spectrometry. Automated data analysis was used to process relative intensities of different glycoforms.

Some chemical modifications are difficult to identify by IEX-HPLC. For example, aspartic acid isomerization or disulfide bond scrambling does not change the charge or charge distribution of a protein and therefore needs to be detected by other techniques. Mass spectrometry-based methods are most sensitive to detect and characterize sequence alterations in proteins. But complex procedures for sample preparation coupled with chromatographic separation and tedious data analysis make mass spectrometry (MS) not very suitable for high-throughput analysis. However, several approaches exist to increase the throughput of MS analysis. Sample preparation procedures can be automated with the help of liquid-handling systems such as those manufactured by companies such as Tecan, Eppendorf, and others. Automated sample preparation is especially beneficial for peptide mapping experiments, which comprise time-consuming sample preparation procedures. Automated procedures have been performed on multi-well plates using the TECAN Evo 100 platform. Some steps of this process are easy to be further simplified. For example, microwave ovens have been used to accelerate the reduction, unfolding, and alkylation reactions [72]. The automated plate-based TriVersa NanoMate autosampler has been introduced by Advion Biosciences (Ithaca, New York) to collect fractions after chromatographic separation for mass analysis by mass spectrometry [73]. The option of multiple injections from a single sample volume increases the accuracy of MS measurements and liberates the analysis from some limitations in chromatographic separation. In some cases, the extremely high resolution and accuracy of modern mass spectrometers allow analysts to abandon chromatographic separation altogether. The method of direct infusion has been described in several studies on glycan analysis [74] and peptide mapping [75]. The combination of these techniques with advanced data analysis creates a perfect foundation for a high-throughput platform for screening of chemical degradations. Using theoretical data on the most probable degradation "hot spots" and pathways, formulation properties and stress conditions should be designed accordingly to confirm or reject the stability predictions. New modifications can be found during analysis and might require reengineering along with additional formulation development. As we have discussed here, analytical techniques which are considered to be low throughput are amenable for being developed into higher throughput techniques, which facilitate automation of sample preparation, analysis of multiple samples by multiple analysis types, and faster analysis times. Another example of such a technique is nuclear magnetic resonance (NMR). NMR has the reputation of being complicated, laborious, and time consuming. However recent technological advances and improvements in automation, sensitivity, resolution, and spectral processing made it is possible to apply NMR for fast and especially very accurate characterization of biopharmaceutical products [76].

We have summarized some of the most common high-throughput analytical methods used in early formulation development in Table 2.1.

2.4 Engineering or formulating protein stability

When drug candidates and formulations are screened for the best desired properties, the question to be asked is whether the inherent stability of the lead-candidate molecule is sufficient for commercialization or significant development is required at later stages to achieve the stability required for a commercial drug product. In some cases, it is possible to reengineer a molecule with greater stable or solubility or both [80,81]. Methods of protein engineering are available to modify the structure of proteins in order to improve stability without compromising biological activity. The biggest challenge of reengineering a protein is to properly understand the correct correlation between the introduced changes in structural properties and protein stability. Empirical approaches that collect stability data on structurally modified molecules can be a good starting point for learning to understand what structural properties relate to greater stability of a biopharmaceutical product. Combined with computational approaches the resulting data sets provide insights to facilitate a decision on whether the stability of a candidate molecule can be improved directly by reengineering or indirectly by formulation development. The more information about a molecule's stability properties is available, the better are the chances to improve its manufacturability and shelf life. mAbs, one of the most common biopharmaceutical modalities, have very similar structural features and properties. Their primary sequences in large parts are fairly well conserved. Yet, due to its ability to recognize and bind to a unique part of hugely diverse foreign targets (antigens), antibodies are diverse by nature as well because of the high sequence variation that exists in the CDR of the Fab (antigen binding) region. Such variety in sequences can lead to difficult development challenges. General

Table 2.1 **High-throughput methods for formulation characterization used in early stages of biopharmaceutical formulation development**

Quality attribute	Methods	Characteristics	References
Conformational stability	Nuclear magnetic resonance (NMR)	Conformation	[20]
	Turbidity	Aggregation propensity	[18]
	Size-exclusion ultra-performance liquid chromatography (SE-UPLC)	Aggregation propensity, fragmentation	[77]
	Dynamic light scattering (DLS)	Aggregation propensity	[49,37]
	Fluorescence	Conformation, aggregation	[17]
	Differential scanning fluorimetry (DSF)	Conformational stability	[15,16]
	Differential scanning calorimetry (DSC)	Conformational stability	[12]
	Precipitation/ solubility	Colloidal stability	[51]
Colloidal stability	Static light scattering (SLS)	Aggregation	[19]
	Ion-exchange ultra-performance liquid chromatography (IEX-UPLC)	Aggregation, charge variants	[76]
	Reversed-phase ultra-performance liquid chromatography (RP-UPLC)	Fragmentation	[75]
	Dynamic light scattering (DLS)	Aggregation, colloidal stability	[73,58]
	Dynamic light scattering (DLS)	Viscosity	[78,79]
	Mass spectrometry	Chemical modifications	[80–82]
Chemical modifications	Ion-exchange ultra-performance liquid chromatography (IEX-UPLC)	Charge modifications	[58]
	Electrophoresis	Charge modifications	[59,60]
	Capillary electrophoresis, fluorescence	Glycopeptide characterization	[70,71]
	Mass spectrometry	Glycopeptide characterization	[74]
Viscosity	Cone and plate	Viscosity, shear rate	[37,47]
	Falling ball	Viscosity by kinetics	[38]
	Capillary, UV imaging	Viscosity by time of migration	[41]
	Capillary, fluorescence	Viscosity by time of migration	[41]
	Dynamic light scattering (DLS)	Viscosity by diffusion coefficient	[44]

stability engineering strategies are complicated by the sequence diversity of an antibody's CDR. Chemical instability of antibodies associated with degradation "hot spots" can be mitigated by eliminating a residue by either replacing it with a more stable residue or complete deletion. Compared to chemical stability, conformational and colloidal stability are more difficult to predict and control. Sequence analysis is still limited in its ability to predict solubility and colloidal stability, which makes the engineering of proteins with improved in-solution properties very difficult. However, some progress has been made in the area of structural design of conformationally and colloidally stable proteins. In the reviews by Rouet et al. and Wu et al., recent advances in the development of aggregation resistant antibody therapeutics are discussed [82,83]. The methods of sequence-based stability predictions are progressively getting better with greater computational power and deeper understanding of the physicochemical mechanisms that influence structural dynamics and conformational stability. One example of complex computational analyses is the research by Davey and Chica, in which the accuracy of predicting the conformational stability of proteins has been improved by multistate computational protein design [84]. In this design, backbone ensembles are used to approximate conformational flexibility, which predict sequence stability with greater quality than predictions using single-state design with a single fixed backbone. In the process of rationalizing the thermodynamics of protein folding, evolutionary theory can be of help [84]. As protein thermodynamics is founded on the statistical mechanics in the space of protein structures, molecular evolution is considered an application in statistical physics and can be viewed as the statistical mechanics in the space of protein sequences. The evolutionary selection of stability of the folded against the unfolded state works better for larger proteins with longer sequences. Another computational approach has been applied in the study of commercially available bevacizumab (Avastin, Genentech/Roche), an angiogenesis inhibitor that slows the growth of new blood vessels. A three-dimensional model of this humanized mAb helped to identify the dimer interface between two bevacizumab molecules [85]. To prevent formation of dimers and the subsequent formation of larger aggregates, docking simulations of different corticosteroids have indicated candidates with the lowest tendency to dimerize. The docking procedure revealed that the preferred interaction occurs between the phosphate group of dexamethasone and the Lys 445 residue of bevacizumab. The structure-based prediction of the inhibitory model was confirmed by in vitro experiments on aggregation propensity under stress conditions in the presence of corticosteroids. In addition to introducing specific mutations, polymer-protein conjugation is applicable to improve molecular stability and solubility. The most common polymer for conjugation is PEG with various molecular weights. The particle formation in egg white lysozyme solutions was analyzed and compared with the conjugated lysozyme molecule diPEG-lysozyme [86] under conditions that involved stresses a protein is commonly exposed to during purification and manufacturing processes. Mechanical agitation, the presence of silicone oil, and freeze–thaw cycling were used to evaluate the aggregation propensity of the native and the conjugated lysozyme. It was found that although the thermal stability of diPEG-lysozyme was lower than for native lysozyme, the overall replacement of attractive protein–protein interactions with repulsive forces reduced the level of particulation. Interestingly, the PEGylated lysozyme absorbed faster onto silicone oil than non-PEGylated lysozyme. The conjugation of external entities to protein molecules should be done along careful analysis of possible changes of structural and colloidal properties caused by such conjugation. PEGylation has been considered to have low impact on immunogenicity. However, recent studies have indicated that the formation of antibodies against the PEG moiety itself is possible. Therefore, the replacement of methoxy-PEG by hydroxyl-PEG for conjugation can provide a safety advantage [87,88]. Other types of conjugation can be provided by several alternatives to PEG. The most advanced alternatives are based on poly(2-oxazoline) [89]. The poly(2-oxazoline) polymers are created by the so called living nature polymerization method. This method allows the synthesis of well-defined block copolymers and variation of the substituent on the 2-position of the 2-oxazoline ring can significantly change the properties of the resulting poly(2-oxazoline)s from hydrophilic (methyl or ethyl) to hydrophobic (longer alkyl or aromatic). These variation possibilities make the class of poly(2-oxazoline)s very well suited for the synthesis of well-defined systematic libraries of (co)polymers and, thus, for the determination of structure–property relationships. Some poly(2-oxazoline) copolymers were also found to increase the uptake of conjugated proteins into cells.

Other approaches to enhance formulation and pharmacokinetic/pharmacodynamic properties of therapeutic proteins include the increase of their half-life by fusing the active protein with the Fc domain of IgG mAbs [90]. In this type of conjugation, the neonatal Fc receptor recycling pathway is utilized to improve not only circulation time but also overall drug stability both in vitro and in vivo [91,92]. The biotherapeutic etanercept (Enbrel, Amgen Inc.) has been developed as a product that is a genetic fusion between the tumor necrosis factor receptor and the Fc domain of a monoclonal antibody. Currently, there are a number of Fc fusion drug candidates at different stages of development, including candidates with modifications to the Fc domain that lead to an enhancement of the antibody-dependent cellular cytotoxicity (ADCC) effector function. A heterodimeric Fc format, with different mutations in the same position of two Fc chains, has been selected by the high-throughput competition AlphaLISA assay for binding activity to FcγRIIIA [93]. As a result, a panel of novel Fc variants was identified with increased ADCC activity in vitro and strong tumor growth inhibition in mice xenograft human models. Specifically a fucosylation of Fc variants further increases the binding of the Fc domain to FcγRIIIA and ADCC activity. And although the stability of the C_H2 region of the modified Fc domains was decreased, the variants remained sufficiently thermodynamically stable for commercialization. Therefore, this work is a good example of complex engineering, which both enhances functional properties and drug product stability. Alternatively, albumin instead of an antibody's Fc domain is used as another option to improve the half-life of therapeutic proteins, and several other recombinant fusion proteins are at various stages of development by pharmaceutical and biopharmaceutical companies [78,79,94].

Any modification to a protein requires careful analysis of potentially incurred structural changes. Whenever possible, molecular modeling should be performed to estimate the effect of introduced nonnative residues on the structural integrity of the protein and consequently to potential changes in protein–protein interactions and protein–solvent properties. The composition and properties of the modified protein's formulation can be very different to that of the native protein. Based on our own experience, many mutations alternate the structural properties of mAbs, which in turn result in both lower conformational and colloidal stability compared with original mAb molecule, and in worst case scenarios to the loss of biological activity. In cases, when the stability is much lower than typically expected for a class of proteins, formulation screening for those proteins should be performed considering a wide range of conditions. Formulation components and properties such as excipients, detergents, pH, and ionic strength can create a stable formulation space that is quite different from that typically observed within a class of proteins.

In many cases the engineering of structural modifications to increase drug product stability is not possible for legal reasons or because the required mutations, additions, and deletions decrease or completely abolish bioactivity. It is not uncommon that the only candidate with sufficient bioactivity is tainted with low solubility or high viscosity. Due to the time constraints commonly experienced in the competitive biopharmaceutical industry, high-throughput formulation screening has become an invaluable tool for the development of stable formulations, in particular for proteins with less than optimal solubility and conformational stability.

On the other hand, if hundreds of suitable, high affinity candidates are available for selecting the most suitable candidate for development and commercialization, screening studies can be specifically designed to identify the most stable of candidates. In those cases, a single formulation can be used under stability decreasing conditions. This "tough" screening approach can be applied to select the "fittest" or most stable molecules. The combination of different stress conditions such as storage at high temperatures, in formulations with a low pH, and in the presence of salt, can be very helpful to remove the less stable proteins from the pool of candidates. At this early stage of development the elimination of the least stable candidates is a priority. However, if the pool of candidates is only comprised of 10–20 molecules, a more careful approach is necessary. A formulation space comprised of the scales of pH, salt concentration, and different excipients can be created in a matrix screening design, in which several stress conditions are applied separately to each candidate to better understand the individual stability profiles. Instead of being eliminated, the candidates should be ranked based on their stability profiles to provide flexibility to the selection process, which may include other criteria than just conformational or colloidal stability or both; e.g., biological activity.

Protein solubility and other types of physicochemical stabilities can be significantly improved by a properly developed formulation during downstream development. However, if even after thorough formulation development, a candidate or a pool of candidates has insufficient stability and solubility properties, a decision should be made on whether to genetically reengineer these candidate(s) to avoid challenges and delays during commercial product development or whether development should be continued, being fully aware of the risk that further formulation development may not be sufficient to commercialize a drug product. Obviously, this decision is highly dependent on the data available, their quality, and how well they address a molecule's liabilities and point to potential solutions.

2.5 Formulation by design

The development of liquid formulations for biotherapeutics has its challenges to stabilize proteins or peptides that never were designed by nature to be stable for a long period of time or soluble at high protein concentrations. In vivo, the majority of biopharmaceuticals has a relatively short half-life in their active form. Usually commercial drug products require a stable shelf life of 1–2 years to be economically viable.

The most commonly recommended temperature for drug product storage is between 2°C and 8°C. However, to increase the accessibility of biopharmaceutical medicines in countries with warm and humid climates that cannot afford the infrastructure to store and handle biologics under cooled conditions, drug product development is trending towards formulations that are stable at ambient temperatures ranging between 25°C and 40°C. To investigate the limits of formulation stability, multiple stress-inducing conditions exist to test and trigger different types of degradation pathways; e.g., high-to-low temperature cycling, sample agitation to simulate transportation, as well as sample handling and transfer. To achieve greater efficacy and more favorable pharmacokinetics for a longer half-life, high-dose product formulations require higher and higher protein concentrations. At the same time, drug product formulations should maintain low viscosity for robust filter and fill-finish operations, as well as drug delivery routes through narrow needle syringes and infusion pumps to decrease the level of pain and increase the level of convenience. As described in the following paragraph, proper formulation design can enable the development of drug product dosage forms that comply with these types of requirements. And as described earlier, automated high-throughput technologies can accelerate the development and execution of the formulation design to frame a formulation design space that comprises the required stability for given formulation requirements.

Fundamental laws of physics determine the behavior of proteins in solutions. Physicists and Biophysical Chemists have employed theories to explain the interactions between proteins and different solution components such as salt, excipients, and other buffer components [94]. The majority of modern liquid biopharmaceutical formulations are a mixture of various molecules with different sizes, charge distributions, and geometries. It is possible to design specific solute molecules that upon addition increase the solubility and stability of specific proteins in their respective formulation solution. Some of these designed excipients are known for enhancing solubility and delivery properties of small molecules. Cyclodextrin-based derivatives, for example, can have hydrophobic, hydrophilic, and ionic properties in solution, and their interaction with small molecules and proteins can be tuned to meet required stability or deliverability criteria [95]. Cyclodextrin appears to be a very useful base molecule to create cyclodextrin-based derivatives with specific properties that enhance the stability of protein and peptide formulations [77,96]. Cyclodextrins significantly increases the solubility of cyclosporine A, a peptide that is almost insoluble in water. In addition, absorption of insulin on the surface of containers is prevented by the addition of cyclodextrin. Branched cyclodextrins are very effective in decreasing the aggregation propensity of recombinant human growth hormone and insulin. The aluminum salt of cyclodextrin is helpful in the prolonged release of basic fibroblast factor. Cyclodextrin derivatives, polymers, and conjugates have been evaluated for practical uses in formulation and drug delivery development. The combination of structural modeling and chemical engineering of excipients can provide the basis for formulation design that is specific to increasing a drug candidate's stability. New technologies for protein delivery pose significant challenges for formulation development. Microsphere- and nanosphere-based technologies provide controlled release under specific formulation conditions, such as pH, buffer, and excipient components. In some cases new delivery systems are coupled with new routes of administration, such as via transdermal, oral, pulmonary, or ocular delivery [97]. Each delivery strategy has its advantages and disadvantages. Selecting the right formulation design, however, should allow to overcome many of the biological and physical constraints [98,99]. In many cases new devices such as autoinjectors or transdermal patches [100] can enhance and improve the quality of delivery. Commercial microfluidic-based implantable patches and pumps [100,101] deliver protein and peptide formulations continuously or by some preprogrammed schedule with high precision. The light weight and convenience of these patches and pumps allow the patients to wear them on their skin and are responsible for their wide use in clinical trials [102–104]. The development of formulations suitable for the use of wearable pumps has some inherent challenges. One of them is the exposure to various surfaces and the increased risk of contamination, which requires the addition of preservatives to maintain sterility. Other challenges involve the exposure to shear that is caused by pistons, rotors, or other moving pump parts. Surfactants or excipients or both can be added to mitigate possible degradation pathways that are induced by protein interactions with surfaces and exposure to shear related stress.

Another relatively new route of biopharmaceutical delivery is pulmonary administration. Studies have shown that compact devices can deliver insulin in the form of an aerosol by inhalation [105]. Aerosol formulations, as a route of delivery, are interesting. Due to the large surface of the aerosol droplets, protein is easily absorbed on the interfaces of different biological tissues.

The number and types of excipients that are accepted for pharmaceutical and biopharmaceutical formulations and their administration is regulated by the regulatory authorities. Any new stabilizer requires extensive testing to comply with regulatory safety requirements. That is why approved excipients should be the preferred first choice in formulation development, and only in cases when the established repertoire of excipients is exhausted and do not provide the required results, the use of nonapproved excipients or the de novo design of new excipient molecules with new desired properties should be considered. However, if the results justify this kind of investment and a new excipient receives regulatory approval, its use for new drug development can provide a significant return of investment, if these excipients are providing benefits in a broader application for a class of molecules.

References

[1] A.S. Rosenberg, Effects of protein aggregates: an immunologic perspective, AAPS J. 8 (3) (2006) E501–E507.

[2] V.S. Purohit, C.R. Middaugh, S.V. Balasubramanian, Influence of aggregation on immunogenicity of recombinant human Factor VIII in hemophilia A mice, J. Pharm. Sci. 95 (2) (2006) 358–371.

[3] M.K. Joubert, M. Hokom, C. Eakin, L. Zhou, M. Deshpande, M.P. Baker, et al., Highly aggregated antibody therapeutics can enhance the in vitro innate and late-stage T-cell immune responses, J. Biol. Chem. 287 (30) (2012) 25266–25279.

[4] J.J. McManus, A. Lomakin, O. Ogun, A. Pande, M. Basan, J. Pande, et al., Altered phase diagram due to a single point mutation in human γD-crystallin, Proc. Natl. Acad. Sci. U.S.A. 104 (43) (2007) 16856–16861.

[5] A. Berg, M. Schuetz, F. Dismer, J. Hubbuch, Automated measurement of apparent protein solubility to rapidly assess complex parameter interactions, Food Bioprod. Process. 92 (2) (2014) 133–142.

[6] M.M. McKinney, A. Parkinson, A simple, non-chromatographic procedure to purify immunoglobulins from serum and ascites fluid, J. Immunol. Methods 96 (2) (1987) 271–278.

[7] V. Kumar, N. Dixit, S.N. Singh, D.S. Kalonia, Phase separation of proteins by poly-ethylene glycols: implications in preformulation and early stage formulation development, Am. Pharm. Rev. 14 (7) (2011) 26–33.

[8] T.J. Gibson, K. Mccarty, I.J. Mcfadyen, E. Cash, P. Dalmonte, K.D. Hinds, et al., Application of a high-throughput screening procedure with PEG-induced precipitation to compare relative protein solubility during formulation development with IgG1 monoclonal antibodies, J. Pharm. Sci. 100 (3) (2011) 1009–1021.

[9] O. Annunziata, N. Asherie, A. Lomakin, J. Pande, O. Ogun, G.B. Benedek, Effect of polyethylene glycol on the liquid–liquid phase transition in aqueous protein solutions, Proc. Natl. Acad. Sci. U.S.A. 99 (22) (2002) 14165–14170.

[10] D.D. Banks, R.F. Latypov, R.R. Ketchem, J. Woodard, J.L. Scavezze, C.C. Siska, et al., Native-state solubility and transfer free energy as predictive tools for selecting excipients to include in protein formulation development studies, J. Pharm. Sci. 101 (8) (2012) 2720–2732.

[11] L. Li, A. Kantor, N. Warne, Application of a PEG precipitation method for solubility screening: a tool for developing high protein concentration formulations, Protein Sci. 22 (8) (2013) 1118–1123.

[12] E. De Bernardez Clark, Refolding of recombinant proteins, Curr. Opin. Biotechnol. 9 (2) (1998) 157–163.

[13] D.J. Callahan, B. Stanley, Y. Li, Control of protein particle formation during ultrafiltration/diafiltration through interfacial protection, J. Pharm. Sci. 103 (3) (2014) 862–869.

[14] N. Dixit, K.M. Maloney, D.S. Kalonia, Protein-silicone oil interactions: comparative effect of nonionic surfactants on the interfacial behavior of a fusion protein, Pharm. Res. 30 (7) (2013) 1848–1859.

[15] W. Lee, W. Fon, B.W. Axelrod, M.L. Roukes, High-sensitivity microfluidic calorimeters for biological and chemical applications, Proc. Natl. Acad. Sci. U.S.A. 106 (36) (2009) 15225–15230.

[16] J. Lerchner, A. Wolf, G. Wolf, V. Baier, E. Kessler, M. Nietzsch, et al., A new microfluid chip calorimeter for biochemical applications, Thermochim. Acta 445 (2) (2006) 144–150.

[17] S. Vermeir, B.M. Nicolai, P. Verboven, P. Van Gerwen, B. Baeten, L. Hoflack, et al., Microplate differential calorimetric biosensor for ascorbic acid analysis in food and pharmaceuticals, Anal. Chem. 79 (16) (2007) 6119–6127.
[18] L. Wang, B. Wang, Q. Lin, Demonstration of MEMS-based differential scanning calorimetry for determining thermodynamic properties of biomolecules, Sens. Actuators B 134 (2) (2008) 953–958.
[19] S. Ghaemmaghami, M.C. Fitzgerald, T.G. Oas, A quantitative, high-throughput screen for protein stability, Proc. Natl. Acad. Sci. U.S.A. 97 (15) (2000) 8296–8301.
[20] S. Fiedler, L. Cole, S. Keller, Automated circular dichroism spectroscopy for medium-throughput analysis of protein conformation, Anal. Chem. 85 (3) (2013) 1868–1872.
[21] M.W. Pantoliano, E.C. Petrella, J.D. Kwasnoski, V.S. Lobanov, J. Myslik, E. Graf, et al., High-density miniaturized thermal shift assays as a general strategy for drug discovery, J. Biomol. Screen. 6 (6) (2001) 429–440.
[22] T.W. Geders, K. Gustafson, B.C. Finzel, Use of differential scanning fluorimetry to optimize the purification and crystallization of PLP-dependent enzymes, Acta Crystallogr. Sect. F Struct. Biol. Cryst. Commun. 68 (5) (2012) 596–600.
[23] L. Alekseychyk, C. Su, G.W. Becker, M.J. Treuheit, V.I. Razinkov, High-throughput screening and stability optimization of anti-streptavidin IgG1 and IgG2 formulations, J. Biomol. Screen. 19 (9) (2014) 1290–1301.
[24] F. He, S. Hogan, R.F. Latypov, L.O. Narhi, V.I. Razinkov, High throughput thermostability screening of monoclonal antibody formulations, J. Pharm. Sci. 99 (4) (2010) 1707–1720.
[25] T. Menzen, W. Friess, High-throughput melting-temperature analysis of a monoclonal antibody by differential scanning fluorimetry in the presence of surfactants, J. Pharm. Sci. 102 (2) (2013) 415–428.
[26] T.J. Magliery, J.J. Lavinder, B.J. Sullivan, Protein stability by number: high-throughput and statistical approaches to one of protein science's most difficult problems, Curr. Opin. Chem. Biol. 15 (3) (2011) 443–451.
[27] N.K. Njoya, R.E. Birdsall, M.J. Wirth, Silica colloidal crystals as emerging materials for high-throughput protein electrophoresis, AAPS J. 15 (4) (2013) 962–969.
[28] J.M. Rizzo, S. Shi, Y. Li, A. Semple, J.J. Esposito, S. Yu, et al., Application of a high-throughput relative chemical stability assay to screen therapeutic protein formulations by assessment of conformational stability and correlation to aggregation propensity, J. Pharm. Sci. 104 (5) (2015) 1632–1640.
[29] H. Nishi, R. Mathäs, R. Fürst, G. Winter, Label-free flow cytometry analysis of subvisible aggregates in liquid IgG1 antibody formulations, J. Pharm. Sci. 103 (1) (2014) 90–99.
[30] S. Chen, H. Lau, Y. Brodsky, G.R. Kleemann, R.F. Latypov, The use of native cation-exchange chromatography to study aggregation and phase separation of monoclonal antibodies, Protein Sci. 19 (6) (2010) 1191–1204.
[31] A. Beck, T. Wurch, C. Bailly, N. Corvaia, Strategies and challenges for the next generation of therapeutic antibodies, Nat. Rev. Immunol. 10 (5) (2010) 345–352.
[32] A.L. Nelson, E. Dhimolea, J.M. Reichert, Development trends for human monoclonal antibody therapeutics, Nat. Rev. Drug Discov. 9 (10) (2010) 767–774.
[33] J.M. Reichert, Antibodies to watch in 2010, MAbs 2 (1) (2010) 84.
[34] S. Yadav, T.M. Laue, D.S. Kalonia, S.N. Singh, S.J. Shire, The influence of charge distribution on self-association and viscosity behavior of monoclonal antibody solutions, Mol. Pharm. 9 (4) (2012) 791–802.
[35] B.D. Connolly, C. Petry, S. Yadav, B. Demeule, N. Ciaccio, J.M. Moore, et al., Weak interactions govern the viscosity of concentrated antibody solutions: high-throughput analysis using the diffusion interaction parameter, Biophys. J. 103 (1) (2012) 69–78.

[36] S.N. Singh, S. Yadav, S.J. Shire, D.S. Kalonia, Dipole-dipole interaction in antibody solutions: correlation with viscosity behavior at high concentration, Pharm. Res. 31 (9) (2014) 2549–2558.
[37] N. Inoue, E. Takai, T. Arakawa, K. Shiraki, Arginine and lysine reduce the high viscosity of serum albumin solutions for pharmaceutical injection, J. Biosci. Bioeng. 117 (5) (2014) 539–543.
[38] S. Yadav, S.J. Shire, D.S. Kalonia, Factors affecting the viscosity in high concentration solutions of different monoclonal antibodies, J. Pharm. Sci. 99 (12) (2010) 4812–4829.
[39] T.W. Patapoff, O. Esue, Polysorbate 20 prevents the precipitation of a monoclonal antibody during shear, Pharm. Dev. Technol. 14 (6) (2009) 659–664.
[40] Y. Eguchi, T. Karino, Measurement of rheologic property of blood by a falling-ball blood viscometer, Ann. Biomed. Eng. 36 (4) (2008) 545–553.
[41] R. Rosencranz, S.A. Bogen, Clinical laboratory measurement of serum, plasma, and blood viscosity, Am. J. Clin. Pathol. 125 (Suppl. 1) (2006) S78–S86.
[42] J. Jezek, M. Rides, B. Derham, J. Moore, E. Cerasoli, R. Simler, et al., Viscosity of concentrated therapeutic protein compositions, Adv. Drug Deliv. Rev. 63 (13) (2011) 1107–1117.
[43] A. Lavoisier, J.-M. Schlaeppi, Early developability screen of therapeutic antibody candidates using Taylor dispersion analysis and UV area imaging detection, MAbs 7 (1) (2015) 77–83.
[44] A. Allmendinger, L.H. Dieu, S. Fischer, R. Mueller, H.C. Mahler, J. Huwyler, High-throughput viscosity measurement using capillary electrophoresis instrumentation and its application to protein formulation, J. Pharm. Biomed. Anal. 99 (2014) 51–58.
[45] D.E. Solomon, S.A. Vanapalli, Multiplexed microfluidic viscometer for high-throughput complex fluid rheology, Microfluid. Nanofluid. 16 (4) (2014) 677–690.
[46] M.A. Haidekker, E.A. Theodorakis, Molecular rotors—fluorescent biosensors for viscosity and flow, Org. Biomol. Chem. 5 (11) (2007) 1669–1678.
[47] F. He, G.W. Becker, J.R. Litowski, L.O. Narhi, D.N. Brems, V.I. Razinkov, High-throughput dynamic light scattering method for measuring viscosity of concentrated protein solutions, Anal. Biochem. 399 (1) (2010) 141–143.
[48] K. Schmitz, Introduction to Dynamic Light Scattering by Macromolecules, Elsevier Science, Amsterdam, 2012, ISBN: 9780323140355.
[49] K.C. Bauer, M.T. Schermeyer, J. Seidel, J. Hubbuch, Impact of polymer surface characteristics on the microrheological measurement quality of protein solutions-a tracer particle screening, Int. J. Pharm. 505 (1–2) (2016) 246–254.
[50] I. Singh, E. Themistou, L. Porcar, S. Neelamegham, Fluid shear induces conformation change in human blood protein von Willebrand factor in solution, Biophys. J. 96 (6) (2009) 2313–2320.
[51] B. Eisenhaber, F. Eisenhaber, Prediction of posttranslational modification of proteins from their amino acid sequence: Data Mining Techniques for the Life Sciences, Humana Press, New York, NY, 2010, 365–384.
[52] H. Rangwala, G. Karypis, Introduction to Protein Structure Prediction: Methods and Algorithms, vol. 14, John Wiley & Sons, Hoboken, NJ, 2010.
[53] R. Sanchez, M. Riddle, J. Woo, J. Momand, Prediction of reversibly oxidized protein cysteine thiols using protein structure properties, Protein Sci. 17 (3) (2008) 473–481.
[54] S. Capasso, S. Salvadori, Effect of the three-dimensional structure on the deamidation reaction of ribonuclease A, J. Pept. Res. 54 (5) (1999) 377–382.
[55] S. Niu, L.L. Hu, L.L. Zheng, T. Huang, K.Y. Feng, Y.D. Cai, et al., Predicting protein oxidation sites with feature selection and analysis approach, J. Biomol. Struct. Dyn. 29 (6) (2012) 1154–1162.

[56] J. Song, K. Burrage, Z. Yuan, T. Huber, Prediction of *cis/trans* isomerization in proteins using PSI-BLAST profiles and secondary structure information, BMC Bioinformatics 7 (1) (2006) 124.
[57] L.W. Dick, D. Qiu, R.B. Wong, K.C. Cheng, Isomerization in the CDR2 of a monoclonal antibody: binding analysis and factors that influence the isomerization rate, Biotechnol. Bioeng. 105 (3) (2010) 515–523.
[58] A. Coffey, Practical Advice for High-Throughput Ion Exchange Separations Using Nonporous Particles, GEN, vol. 32, No. 13, 2012.
[59] T.D. Wheeler, J.L. Sun, S. Pleiner, H. Geier, P. Dobberthien, J. Studts, et al., Microchip zone electrophoresis for high throughput analysis of monoclonal antibody charge variants, Anal. Chem. 86 (11) (2014) 5416–5424.
[60] J. Creamer, N.J. Oborny, S.M. Lunte, Recent advances in the analysis of therapeutic proteins by capillary and microchip electrophoresis, Anal. Methods 6 (15) (2014) 5427–5449.
[61] H. Han, E. Livingston, X. Chen, High throughput profiling of charge heterogeneity in antibodies by microchip electrophoresis, Anal. Chem. 83 (21) (2011) 8184–8191.
[62] M.J. Gramer, Product quality considerations for mammalian cell culture process development and manufacturing: Mammalian Cell Cultures for Biologics Manufacturing, Springer Berlin, Heidelberg, 2014, 123–166.
[63] R. Jefferis, Isotype and glycoform selection for antibody therapeutics, Arch. Biochem. Biophys. 526 (2) (2012) 159–166.
[64] R. Jefferis, Glycosylation as a strategy to improve antibody-based therapeutics, Nat. Rev. Drug Discov. 8 (3) (2009) 226–234.
[65] N. Taniguchi, J. Gu, M. Takahashi, E. Miyoshi, Functional glycomics and evidence for gain-and loss-of-functions of target proteins for glycosyltransferases involved in *N*-glycan biosynthesis: their pivotal roles in growth and development, cancer metastasis and antibody therapy against cancer, Proc. Jpn. Acad., Ser. B, Phys. Biol. Sci. 80 (2) (2004) 82–91.
[66] L.N. Robinson, C. Artpradit, R. Raman, Z.H. Shriver, M. Ruchirawat, R. Sasisekharan, Harnessing glycomics technologies: integrating structure with function for glycan characterization, Electrophoresis 33 (5) (2012) 797–814.
[67] S.R. Kronewitter, H.J. An, M.L. de Leoz, C.B. Lebrilla, S. Miyamoto, G.S. Leiserowitz, The development of retrosynthetic glycan libraries to profile and classify the human serum *N*-linked glycome, Proteomics 9 (11) (2009) 2986–2994.
[68] T. Song, S. Ozcan, A. Becker, C.B. Lebrilla, In-depth method for the characterization of glycosylation in manufactured recombinant monoclonal antibody drugs, Anal. Chem. 86 (12) (2014) 5661–5666.
[69] D.A. Shepherd, M.T. Marty, K. Giles, A.J. Baldwin, J.L. Benesch, Combining tandem mass spectrometry with ion mobility separation to determine the architecture of polydisperse proteins, Int. J. Mass Spectrom. (2014). http://dx.doi.org/10.1016/j.ijms.2014.09.007.
[70] C. Váradi, C. Lew, A. Guttman, Rapid magnetic bead based sample preparation for automated and high throughput *N*-glycan analysis of therapeutic antibodies, Anal. Chem. 86 (12) (2014) 5682–5687.
[71] D. Reusch, M. Haberger, M.H. Selman, P. Bulau, A.M. Deelder, M. Wuhrer, et al., High-throughput work flow for IgG Fc-glycosylation analysis of biotechnological samples, Anal. Biochem. 432 (2) (2013) 82–89.
[72] P.M. Reddy, Y.S. Huang, C.T. Chen, P.C. Chang, Y.P. Ho, Evaluating the potential non-thermal microwave effects of microwave-assisted proteolytic reactions, J. Proteomics 80 (2013) 160–170.

[73] M. Lorenz, O.S. Ovchinnikova, G.J. Van Berkel, Fully automated laser ablation liquid capture surface analysis using nanoelectrospray ionization mass spectrometry, Rapid Commun. Mass Spectrom. 28 (11) (2014) 1312–1320.
[74] J.M. Prien, B.D. Prater, Q. Qin, S.L. Cockrill, Mass spectrometric-based stable isotopic 2-aminobenzoic acid glycan mapping for rapid glycan screening of biotherapeutics, Anal. Chem. 82 (4) (2010) 1498–1508.
[75] A. Lu, L.F. Waanders, R. Almeida, G. Li, M. Allen, J. Cox, et al., Nanoelectrospray peptide mapping revisited: composite survey spectra allow high dynamic range protein characterization without LCMS on an orbitrap mass spectrometer, Int. J. Mass Spectrom. 268 (2) (2007) 158–167.
[76] D.S. Wishart, Characterization of biopharmaceuticals by NMR spectroscopy, Trends Anal. Chem. 48 (2013) 96–111.
[77] M.E. Brewster, M.S. Hora, J.W. Simpkins, N. Bodor, Use of 2-hydroxypropyl-β-cyclodextrin as a solubilizing and stabilizing excipient for protein drugs, Pharm. Res. 8 (6) (1991) 792–795.
[78] M.A. Bush, J.E. Matthews, E.H. De Boever, R.L. Dobbins, R.J. Hodge, S.E. Walker, et al., Safety, tolerability, pharmacodynamics and pharmacokinetics of albiglutide, a long-acting glucagon-like peptide-1 mimetic, in healthy subjects, Diabetes Obes. Metab. 11 (5) (2009) 498–505.
[79] E. Santagostino, C. Negrier, R. Klamroth, A. Tiede, I. Pabinger-Fasching, C. Voigt, et al., Safety and pharmacokinetics of a novel recombinant fusion protein linking coagulation factor IX with albumin (rIX-FP) in hemophilia B patients, Blood 120 (12) (2012) 2405–2411.
[80] C. Ó'Fágáin, Engineering protein stability: Protein Chromatography, Humana Press, New York, NY, 2011, 103–136.
[81] J. Maynard, G. Georgiou, Antibody engineering, Ann. Rev. Biomed. Eng. 2 (1) (2000) 339–376.
[82] R. Rouet, D. Lowe, D. Christ, Stability engineering of the human antibody repertoire, FEBS Lett. 588 (2) (2014) 269–277.
[83] S.J. Wu, J. Luo, K.T. O'Neil, J. Kang, E.R. Lacy, G. Canziani, et al., Structure-based engineering of a monoclonal antibody for improved solubility, Protein Eng. Des. Sel. 23 (8) (2010) 643–651.
[84] J.A. Davey, R.A. Chica, Improving the accuracy of protein stability predictions with multistate design using a variety of backbone ensembles, Proteins 82 (5) (2014) 771–784.
[85] M. Veurink, Y. Westermaier, R. Gurny, L. Scapozza, Breaking the aggregation of the monoclonal antibody bevacizumab (Avastin®) by dexamethasone phosphate: insights from molecular modelling and asymmetrical flow field-flow fractionation, Pharm. Res. 30 (4) (2013) 1176–1187.
[86] L.S. Holm, A. Mcumber, J.E. Rasmussen, M. Obiols-Rabasa, P.W. Thulstrup, M.R. Kasimova, et al., The effect of protein PEGylation on physical stability in liquid formulation, J. Pharm. Sci. 103 (10) (2014) 3043–3054.
[87] M.R. Sherman, L.D. Williams, M.A. Sobczyk, S.J. Michaels, M.G. Saifer, Role of the methoxy group in immune responses to mPEG-protein conjugates, Bioconjug. Chem. 23 (3) (2012) 485–499.
[88] M.G. Saifer, L.D. Williams, M.A. Sobczyk, S.J. Michaels, M.R. Sherman, Selectivity of binding of PEGs and PEG-like oligomers to anti-PEG antibodies induced by methoxyPEG-proteins, Mol. Immunol. 57 (2) (2014) 236–246.

[89] J. Tong, R. Luxenhofer, X. Yi, R. Jordan, A.V. Kabanov, Protein modification with amphiphilic block copoly (2-oxazoline)s as a new platform for enhanced cellular delivery, Mol. Pharm. 7 (4) (2010) 984–992.
[90] T. Suzuki, A. Ishii-Watabe, M. Tada, T. Kobayashi, T. Kanayasu-Toyoda, T. Kawanishi, et al., Importance of neonatal FcR in regulating the serum half-life of therapeutic proteins containing the Fc domain of human IgG1: a comparative study of the affinity of monoclonal antibodies and Fc-fusion proteins to human neonatal FcR, J. Immunol. 184 (4) (2010) 1968–1976.
[91] N.J. Boylan, W. Zhou, R.J. Proos, T.J. Tolbert, J.L. Wolfe, J.S. Laurence, Conjugation site heterogeneity causes variable electrostatic properties in Fc conjugates, Bioconjug. Chem. 24 (6) (2013) 1008–1016.
[92] T. Rath, K. Baker, J.A. Dumont, R.T. Peters, H. Jiang, S.W. Qiao, et al., Fc-fusion proteins and FcRn: structural insights for longer-lasting and more effective therapeutics, Crit. Rev. Biotechnol. (2013) 1–20. http://dx.doi.org/10.3109/07388551.2013.834293.
[93] Z. Liu, K. Gunasekaran, W. Wang, V. Razinkov, L. Sekirov, E. Leng, et al., Asymmetrical Fc engineering greatly enhances antibody-dependent cellular cytotoxicity (ADCC) effector function and stability of the modified antibodies, J. Biol. Chem. 289 (6) (2014) 3571–3590.
[94] S. Schulte, Innovative coagulation factors: albumin fusion technology and recombinant single-chain factor VIII, Thromb. Res. 131 (2013) S2–S6.
[95] K. Uekama, Design and evaluation of cyclodextrin-based drug formulation, Chem. Pharm. Bull. 52 (8) (2004) 900–915.
[96] R. Challa, A. Ahuja, J. Ali, R.K. Khar, Cyclodextrins in drug delivery: an updated review, AAPS PharmSciTech 6 (2) (2005) E329–E357.
[97] S. Mitragotri, P.A. Burke, R. Langer, Overcoming the challenges in administering biopharmaceuticals: formulation and delivery strategies, Nat. Rev. Drug Discov. 13 (2014) 655–672.
[98] H. Lennernäs, Intestinal permeability and its relevance for absorption and elimination, Xenobiotica 37 (10–11) (2007) 1015–1051.
[99] P.W. Wertz, Current understanding of skin biology pertinent to skin penetration: skin biochemistry, Skin Pharmacol. Physiol. 26 (4–6) (2013) 217–226.
[100] M.R. Prausnitz, R. Langer, Transdermal drug delivery, Nat. Biotechnol. 26 (11) (2008) 1261–1268.
[101] L. Ricotti, T. Assaf, P. Dario, A. Menciassi, Wearable and implantable pancreas substitutes, J. Artif. Organs 16 (1) (2013) 9–22.
[102] P. Schaepelynck, P. Darmon, L. Molines, M.F. Jannot-Lamotte, C. Treglia, D. Raccah, Advances in pump technology: insulin patch pumps, combined pumps and glucose sensors, and implanted pumps, Diabetes Metab. 37 (2011) S85–S93.
[103] A.C.R. Grayson, I.S. Choi, B.M. Tyler, P.P. Wang, H. Brem, M.J. Cima, et al., Multi-pulse drug delivery from a resorbable polymeric microchip device, Nat. Mater. 2 (11) (2003) 767–772.
[104] R. Farra, N.F. Sheppard, L. McCabe, R.M. Neer, J.M. Anderson, J.T. Santini, et al., First-in-human testing of a wirelessly controlled drug delivery microchip, Sci. Transl. Med. 4 (122) (2012). 122ra21.
[105] H. Zisser, L. Jovanovic, K. Markova, R. Petrucci, A. Boss, P. Richardson, et al., Technosphere insulin effectively controls postprandial glycemia in patients with type 2 diabetes mellitus, Diabetes Technol. Ther. 14 (11) (2012) 997–1001.

Preclinical and clinical formulation studies

3

3.1 High-throughput manufacturability assessment

From the initial pool of molecule candidates, only a few, usually 5–10, molecules are selected for an assessment of their manufacturability. The intent of this assessment is to identify the one candidate that is most suitable to be manufactured at clinical and commercial scale. To this end, the candidates are exposed and tested under conditions that closely resemble those during manufacturing, storage, and delivery. Conditions mimicking the human physiology should be tested as well to investigate the drug candidate's in vivo stability in the human body. Formulation screening is an important part of creating a stable drug product that is suited for clinical and commercial manufacture. If the pool of lead candidates is small and the available amount of protein is relatively large, a wide range of formulations and conditions can be investigated using a wide range of different analytical methods. If the class of protein entering the molecule assessment is well known and characterized, the initial screening of formulation conditions can be more directed and defined. For example, monoclonal antibodies (mAbs) have been a focus of development in the biopharmaceutical industry for more than two decades. Suitable antibody formulations have been developed and proven to be stable for a number of different commercial products. As a result, formulation platforms with common buffer types, excipients, and pH values have been developed and applied for clinical and commercial antibody development. However, even well-developed and characterized formulation platforms require in many instances additional product-specific optimization and refinement to produce a manufacturable drug product. One-fits-all formulations are hard to find, even for molecule classes with high structural similarity. Platform formulations serve well in accelerating lead-candidate development for Phase 1 and Phase 2 clinical studies. Nevertheless, more often than not, further development and refinement is necessary for Phase 3 clinical studies and commercialization. For non-platform candidates, because of a lesser understanding of the molecular properties and stability, formulation screening should comprise a wide range of formulation compositions and properties. The early assessment of molecular properties can save resources and development time for purification process, commercial formulation, and analytical method development.

During the phase of candidate selection and manufacturability assessment, only limited knowledge exists about in how far protein degradation products impact the potency and safety of a protein drug candidate. The lack of toxicity data and clinical results complicate the selection of appropriate methods and analytics that suitably mimic conditions, material contacts, and shear forces during drug production and delivery to educate the selection of the top candidates for clinical development. At this stage, the amount of purified product is rather limited, which in turn limits the number

High-Throughput Formulation Development of Biopharmaceuticals. DOI: http://dx.doi.org/10.1016/B978-1-907568-63-3.00003-7

of samples and assays that can be conducted during manufacturability assessment. High-throughput methodologies can significantly improve the amount of information that is needed to be gained by being able to handle many samples of small volumes in a short period of time, while at the same time consuming only little amounts of protein. Furthermore, to take full advantage of high-throughput studies, it is important to select methods and assays that assess the relevant factors that well represent drug substance and drug product processes during upstream and downstream processing. The primary question associated with formulation screening is how adequate and relevant the simulating stresses are to the production of a biotherapeutic. Obviously there are a number of stress conditions associated with manufacturing of biopharmaceuticals. During the upstream process the protein can degrade or become chemically modified in cell culture (posttranslational modifications) and the protein solution can contain cell-based or product-based impurities. The protein purification process is designed to remove those impurities and degradation products. However, the process of purification also introduces stress conditions, like low-pH viral inactivation, that may induce protein degradation.

The purification of biopharmaceutical products includes several chromatography steps, viral inactivation at low pH, and filtration under different conditions [1]. Ion-exchange chromatography is an important step in the purification process and the conditions and contact with the column resin on a separation column can induce stress on the protein structure. Cation-exchange (CEX) chromatography can increase the aggregation level of mAbs, possibly because of the high concentration of salt present in the mobile phase or interaction with the column resin or both [2].

For biopharmaceutical drugs produced in animal or plant cells, viral deactivation and clearance to very low acceptable levels is typically required. Some level of viral clearance is achieved during purification by chromatography, but additional steps may be required to inactivate and to sufficiently remove the remaining viral content. For example, during the purification process of mAbs, viral inactivation at low pH between pH 3.0 and pH 4.0, and virus removal by filtration are employed. High-aggregation propensity caused by decreased conformational stability at low pH during the viral inactivation step can induce a problem for maintaining sufficient protein stability and activity for the subsequent purification steps and overall yield of natively folded, active and stable protein [3]. Under low pH conditions, in some cases, the unfolding temperature can drop all the way to ambient temperature. In combination with high ionic strength, conformational stability can be further reduced. Therefore, the formulation study design for manufacturability should include a wide range of pH values and salt concentrations to evaluate the limits of acceptable solution conditions. The most common limiting factor during early development of protein candidates is poor solubility. During downstream process development, characterization of solution stability is important to be prepared for the many steps of protein processing such as inclusion body refolding, chromatography, and filtration. High-throughput methods for rapid solubility screening have been used to assess the apparent solubility of lysozyme [4]. Various parameters were used to optimize protein solubility. Ionic strength, pH, and excipient concentration, as well as various combinations were tested for statistical significance and interactions between them. It was found that pH and temperature act in a statistically significant two-way interaction on protein stability, and that there is significant influence of ionic strength on the additive-induced changes in apparent solubility. At the high salt concentrations lysozyme solubility have been improved in the presence of polyethylene glycols (PEGs) and polysorbate 20. This approach was shown to be helpful to understand the mechanism of lysozyme aggregation and to accurately map the relevant formulation space for high solubility.

Different filtration processes also play an essential part in purifying pharmaceutical grade proteins. Viral removal may include filtration through filters with pore sizes less than 20 nm [5]. Filtration-induced stresses associated with shear forces, pressure, and concentration gradients, especially with high-viscosity formulations, can cause conformational changes or the protein to aggregate on the surface of a filter [6]. In addition to the challenges during manufacturing and purification, transportation, storage, and delivery processes may incur further strain on the structural integrity of a biotherapeutic, which should be also evaluated in manufacturability assessment studies. To this end, manufacturability assessment studies of protein drug formulations are conducted under conditions that mimic the manufacture, storage, and delivery-induced stresses. These include storage conditions at elevated temperatures above the recommended storage temperature, exposure to light, freeze–thaw cycling, and the contact with different surfaces. Proteins are susceptible to the ultraviolet spectrum of light, specifically amino acid residues such as tryptophan, tyrosine, phenylalanine, cysteine, and methionine. According to the ICH Q1B guideline, [7] D65 is the internationally recognized standard for outdoor daylight and ID65 is the equivalent indoor indirect daylight standard. Typical photostability studies should be performed by exposing the samples to at least 1.2 lux hours and integrated 200 Wh/m^2. For this type of study, control samples covered by foil should be present in the photochamber. To accelerate degradation, manufacturability assessment photostability studies should be conducted at light intensities much higher than recommended by the ICH guidelines. Frequent photo-induced degradations of antibodies include tryptophan and methionine oxidation, aggregation, and non-reducible thioether crosslinks [8,9]. In light-induced stress studies it is useful to screen for formulations that contain excipients with protective properties against light-induced modifications [10]. In this context, special care has to be taken in high-throughput study setups, especially with plate-based setups, to ensure uniform light exposure of every well on the plate. In addition, the material of the container, whether it is a vial or a plate, should represent as closely as possible the material of the relevant drug product container with identical or closely similar absorbance properties.

Another condition that can put stress on the structural integrity of a drug substance and drug product candidate during storage and delivery is freeze–thaw cycling. For frozen liquid formulations, freeze–thaw cycling represents a normal condition for storing and preparing a biotherapeutic for delivery. The recommended storage temperature for a frozen drug product formulation ranges typically between −20°C and −30°C. Frozen drug substance formulations are typically stored at −30°C. Reference standard is often stored between −70°C and −80°C. Therefore, to account for this wide range of sub-zero temperatures, a typical freeze–thaw study includes five to seven freeze–thaw cycles that are comprised of a 1- to 2-day incubation at either −20°C or −30°C and −70°C that is followed by a complete thawing step at either 2°C to 8°C or controlled room temperature. The preferential formation of ice crystals during freezing is mainly responsible for conformational changes primarily induced at the liquid–ice interface of the ice crystals and solution [11]. In addition, the fraction of the unfrozen liquid may undergo significant changes in solute concentration and pH. Those changes in the physical environment of a protein may lead to precipitation, liquid–liquid phase separation (LLPS) and protein unfolding. For example, during freezing, changes in pH in solutions of phosphates depend on the relative contents of sodium and potassium [12]. Stabilizing agents such as sugars, amino acids, and salts are used to stabilize proteins during the freeze–thaw process [13]. On the other hand, excipients can crystallize or phase-separate during freezing and cause structural damage to proteins either by interactions between the excipient crystals and protein or by the lack of stabilizing interactions between the excipient and the protein because they are separated by different phases [14]. The screening of samples during freeze–thaw cycling should be preferably executed in the same storage containers, ideally made of the same material as the respective drug substance or drug product container, because the surface material of the container plays a role in the overall stability of the protein and crystallization propensity of excipients. Typical degradation pathways include aggregation, precipitation, and phase separation. After freeze–thaw cycling is completed, high-throughput analytical methods can be applied, using a multi-well plate format, to investigate the resulting degradation products. In some cases, especially during early development when material is limited and it is difficult to provide enough protein to execute freeze–thaw studies in full-size drug substance or drug product containers, the use of multi-well plates is justified for quick evaluation of formulation stability that is suitable for preclinical formulation development and toxicology studies. Also for lyophilized formulations it is possible to screen different composition in the plate-based format. A recent study showed that freeze-drying of formulations on multi-well plates resulted in physical properties similar to those obtained in vials [15]. Trnka et al. were able to demonstrate and confirm by high-throughput X-ray powder diffraction that the polymorphic outcome was independent of the container. The expected increase in moisture level, because of the increasing amount of amorphous matter in the samples, was observed in both vials and multi-well plates. The cake structure and properties were adequate in multi-well plates and could be effectively quantified using image analysis. The reconstitution time was also found to be equal in all three platforms (i.e., in brass well plates, plastic well plates, and vials) and no significant edge effect was discovered.

In such cases, when greater amounts of protein are available, the number of analytical techniques and stress-inducing conditions that comprise a formulation screening study can be increased to create more comprehensive and informative data sets during manufacturability assessment, allowing to study both the conformational and colloidal stability of the protein candidates under investigation. As mentioned above, the conformational stability of a protein drug candidate can be determined by measuring its unfolding temperature in a given formulation. In a high-throughput format, this is typically accomplished by using differential scanning fluorimetry (DSF), as described in the previous section. The method is very suitable for the evaluation of multiple formulations with small sample volumes. DSF can be used for protein formulations with protein concentrations ranging from 0.1 to 100 mg/mL. One example is the study of the conformational and colloidal stability of mAbs, tested by DSF and high-throughput differential static light scattering (DSLS) [16]. In this work, the DSLS method used static light scattering (SLS) to evaluate the level of protein stability during thermal denaturation in a 384-well format. Protein aggregation was induced by incubation at elevated temperature (40°C) and analyzed by comparing DSF with DSLS measurements. A SLS plate reader StarGazer-384 (Harbinger Biotechnology and Engineering Corporation, Markham, Ontario, Canada) was used to evaluate the colloidal stability of antibodies at a protein concentration of 1 mg/mL. The intensity of scattered light was measured at 600 nm with 25 μL of the sample heated at 70°C. The lag time before the onset of aggregation was used to screen and optimize the formulations for different excipients. The study showed that the mAb aggregation level is controlled by both conformational and colloidal stability. The implementation of DSF and DSLS high-throughput techniques helped to monitor the conformational and colloidal stability of multiple formulations. The multi-well plate platform used in this study provided an excellent opportunity to screen stabilizing excipients and to differentiate between different concentrations of excipients, as well as the effects of multiple excipients on mAb conformational and colloidal stability. It is worthwhile to note that protein aggregation at high temperatures is typically induced by conformational changes, specifically by partial or complete unfolding. It is more difficult to predict the aggregation propensity of a protein at lower temperatures, when the contribution of conformational stability is negligible and aggregation primarily depends on a protein's colloidal stability. As mentioned before, the presence of unfolded or partially unfolded protein in a formulation solution can result in protein aggregation because of interactions between exposed hydrophobic residues or surface areas that are structurally protected from the solvent and intermolecular interactions between proteins in their fully folded native state. Hydrophobicity-sensitive fluorescence probes such as 1-anilinonaphthalene-8-sulfonate (ANS), 4,4′-bis(1-anilinonaphthalene-8-sulfonate) (bis-ANS), Nile Red, and Congo Red can be used to detect and characterize unfolded and aggregated proteins in a high-throughput format. However, various factors can interfere with the results of those experiments. ANS-based probes have been shown to bind to some proteins through electrostatic interactions [17]. Nile Red and Congo Red can be sensitive to pH and buffer composition [18,19]. Previously, the use of SYPRO Orange was described for DSF measurements to screen the conformational stability of protein formulations. Specifically antibody formulations are very accommodative for this methodology because of the low SYPRO Orange fluorescence background in the presence of native and properly folded mAbs. In our laboratory we used this methodology to detect and quantify the level of stress-induced aggregates in antibody formulations [20]. It was shown that the fluorescence intensity of the dye in the presence of aggregated mAb correlated very well with the level of aggregated mAb measured by traditional analytical size-exclusion high-performance liquid chromatography (SE-HPLC). To increase the throughput of the fluorescence measurements the experiments were carried out on 96-well plates using a fluorescence plate reader. It could be demonstrated that the amount of large particles determined by micro-flow imaging was proportional to the fluorescence intensity of samples with mechanically induced particles. This method is especially attractive for the characterization of highly concentrated formulations, in which the relative percentage of aggregates is typically low. Any analytical method to quantify the amount of aggregated protein at high concentrations requires significant dilution to remain in the linear range of the measurement. The sensitivity of fluorescence-based measurements is directly dependent on the absolute amount of unfolded aggregated protein, with greater sensitivity in higher concentrated protein solutions at the same level of aggregates. The main disadvantage of this technique lies in the difficulty of being able to determine whether or not the measured aggregates are actually comprised of unfolded or folded protein. Native self-association is possible and often reversible, and cannot be detected by the use of fluorescence probes that depend on the exposure and interaction of hydrophobic residues or surface areas. In any case, carefully designed and executed calibration procedures are necessary to measure accurate amounts of aggregates. All things considered, this methodology is useful for fast, small volume, and high content screening studies of protein formulations after incubation at elevated temperatures or other structure impeding types of stresses.

Stress-induced protein degradation products and modifications can be analyzed by various chromatographic methods commonly used in formulation development. Separation techniques like size-exclusion, reversed-phase, ion-exchange, hydrophobic and hydrophilic interaction high-performance liquid chromatography (HPLC) are conventionally low-throughput methods and they require relatively long run times to achieve the necessary peak separation for accurate and reliable quantification. Ultra-high pressure chromatography systems and new generations of resins allow much shorter run times by maintaining the peak resolution of traditional HPLC systems. For example, phenyl columns with a particle size of 1.7 μm have been used in ultra-performance liquid chromatography (UPLC) systems applying reversed-phase chromatography for the analysis of mAb fragmentation [21]. With this setup, the run time could be reduced to 5–10 minutes, which is four to five times shorter than the typical run times of a similar method performed on a lower pressure reversed-phase HPLC system. New resin materials have been introduced to ion-exchange HPLC methods using Bio WCX NP3 (Agilent Technologies Inc., Santa Clara, California) and Bio Pro SP-F (YMC America Inc., Allentown, Pennsylvania) columns for increased throughput applications. The use of pH gradient ion-exchange HPLC has been successfully used for high-resolution charge variant analysis of mAbs [22]. The pH gradients were generated by mixing defined buffer components. The buffer compositions were optimized for several mAbs. The results indicated that a universal method that was optimized for multiple molecules was robust and had a resolution and peak capacity comparable or better than that of ionic-strength elution ion-exchange HPLC. Direct analysis (no buffer exchange) of samples in matrixes consistent with in-process manufacturing pools was demonstrated to perform high-throughput evaluations of in-process and final product samples. Optimized UV-based methods for detection along with high-throughput size-exclusion HPLC methods has improved the analysis of highly concentrated antibody formulations frequently used in clinical development [23]. Changing the detection wavelength from 215 to 235 nm allowed approximately a fivefold increase in injection volume and eliminated the need of dilution of highly concentrated protein samples for analysis.

The propensity of antibody self-association can be screened by a new and improved version of self-interaction nanoparticle spectroscopy (SINS) [24]. The SINS-based methodology is capable of characterizing repulsive and attractive interactions between mAb molecules in solution. Antibodies immobilized on the surface of gold nanoparticles can induce repulsion or attraction between nanoparticles. The distance between particles determines the shift of the plasmon wavelength. This shift is also dependent on the amount of antibody immobilized on the surface and is correlated with diffusion interaction parameters determined at much higher protein concentrations. SINS measurements of various formulations can be performed in a high-throughput, multi-well plate format. In another study the propensity of protein aggregation was evaluated by exposing mAb samples to mechanical stress caused by shaking (agitation) and thermal stress [25]. The high-throughput assessment of protein stability was performed by measuring the temperature of hydrophobic exposure (T_h, thermal stability) and the diffusion interaction parameter (k_D, colloidal stability). Incubation at high temperature resulted in an increase in soluble oligomers while mechanical stress led to increased formation of large particles. To determine the optimal formulation compositions, the study, including the stress methods, was set up on multi-well plates, and the obtained high-throughput data were analyzed by statistical models, which will be discussed in greater detail later.

Automated methodologies also provide greater accuracy and reproducibility of measurements by decreasing human error in liquid handling and measurements. Well maintained and regularly calibrated, automated processes can significantly improve the quality of analytical results [26]. Companies such as Tecan Group Ltd. (Männedorf, Switzerland), Eppendorf (Hamburg, Germany), and Hamilton (Reno, Nevada) provide a line of liquid handling systems that can be used to prepare samples containing both multiple candidates and multiple formulations. The sample volume used in those systems can be as low as a few microliters to handle the small amount of protein usually available during molecule and manufacturability assessment studies. Liquid handling systems can also have various platforms incorporated into an automated process for stress applications and analytical measurements. Such incorporation makes it possible to create continuous workflows that start with the sample preparation and end with a set of analytical data obtained by different assays under different conditions. Various sample holders, available for automation and quick formulation screenings, are reviewed by Majors [27]. High-throughput screening often utilizes a multi-well plate format for sample preparation and handling. The material of the plates and wells is in most cases different from the container or device material used for drug substance and drug product storage and delivery processes. Container and device materials become a critical factor if protein–surface interactions play a significant role in formulation stability. Ideally the plate material is made of the same material as the drug product vials or syringes to ensure that the screening data are representative of the same degradation pathways that occur in the designated drug product container. In addition, the appropriate fill volume and geometry of a given container need to be considered in stability evaluations of a biological drug product. Often, additional studies are recommended to establish comparability of high-throughput screening procedures with the procedures routinely used in process development. Instrumentation, using a 96-well plate-based setup, normally requires only a small amount of material ranging from microliters to a few milliliters. The Society for Laboratory Automation and Screening (SLAS) is providing a roadmap, which is readily adaptable for high-throughput applications [28]. As mentioned before, the multi-well plates used for high-throughput screening may have a surface chemistry, geometry, and other properties that is different from the final drug product container. Formulation screening or any other studies can be affected by protein–surface interactions. The surface effects are less pronounced in quick turnaround screening studies with relatively short incubation times and temperatures between 2°C and 8°C, assuming that the container surface is not reactive. The impact of protein–surface interactions on protein stability can be more significant in long-term stability studies with extended holding periods at room temperature and above. In many cases, storage at low temperature over long periods of time can induce product instabilities by random, slow, and hard-to-predict container material related events such as microcracks formation and leaching of impurities from the container surface. Certain mini-vial insert systems, comparable with the SLAS footprint for 96-well plates, can help to investigate potential container surface and material concerns. The glass vial inserts used in these systems have the same chemical composition and surface characteristics as commonly used borosilicate type 1 glass vials with stoppers made of butyl rubber and Fluro Tec coating. Another solution to simulate drug product vial and syringe materials is to use plates made of the same material; e.g., glass or plastic. However, the issue of adequate container volume to fill volume ratios and container geometry still remain to be addressed.

The next level of instrument development, as well as solution and sample volume miniaturization is the chip-based configuration of analytical- and liquid-handling systems. The Lab-on-a-Chip (LOC) concept has been first introduced in 1980 based on the principles of a gas chromatographic air analyzer [29]. However, it was not until 1990 when the microfabrication technology reached a level of sophistication that made it possible to assemble analysis systems that were comprised of various types of micro pumps, flow sensors, and integrated fluid treatments [30]. The development of Microelectromechanical Systems (MEMS) also contributed significantly to the implementation of LOC technologies for pharmaceutical and biopharmaceutical analyses. The LOC technology has various applications for protein and peptide formulation development. The advantages of LOC applications include improved control of input parameters, small system size, and safer, environmentally friendly studies because of smaller sample and solution volumes, lower energy consumption, and high integration of functionality. The ability of a chip-based setup to easily replicate the included system modules in parallel arrays make the technology adaptable to high-throughput analyses. In such a miniaturized high-throughput system, fast analysis and response time are a result of short flow pathways and high surface to volume ratios. The major disadvantages of the LOC technology are attributed to specific effects that are intrinsic to the chemical and physical properties of small scale designs. Those effects are capillary forces, interactions with surface materials and surface properties (e.g., roughness). Also, the signal-to-noise ratio and the accuracy of the measurements on complex integrated systems can be significantly lower than those on standalone analytical micro- and nanoscale instrumentation. Furthermore, the implementation of LOC technologies for formulation development can face additional obstacles such as high viscosity of concentrated protein solutions, which can prevent liquid from flowing consistently and reliably through the small diameter channels of the chip platform. High surface to volume ratios can enhance the selective absorption of formulation components. Analytical LOC instruments are most commonly comprised of disposable system modules because it is difficult to clean microfabricated channels, chambers, and cells. Therefore, maintaining consistent mechanical parameters and physical properties is very important to preserve the highest possible reproducibility of analytical measurements. An automated Lab-on-a-Chip platform (ALP) was used as a part of a robotic high-throughput laboratory system for the screening of a variety of antibody formulations [31]. In this setup the ALP is a microfluid technology that is used as an alternative to traditional sodium dodecyl sulfate polyacrylamide gel electrophoresis (SDS-PAGE) to separate proteins and protein fragments. To detect protein degradation products, such as protein fragments and aggregates, the protein samples were prepared under both reducing and non-reducing conditions and analyzed automatically on reusable microfluid chips. The separated protein bands were stained with a fluorescence dye, destained and detected by a laser-induced fluorescence detector. The total time to complete the experiment takes less than a minute. LOC technologies are still a relatively new platform for the biopharmaceutical industry and more development is required to incorporate chip-based systems more routinely into the processes of formulation preparation and characterization. For the near future it is expected that integrated miniaturized chip-based platforms will be commonly used to monitor real-time drug product stability without the need of separate unit operations for sample preparation and measurements. Especially in the early phases of formulation development when optimal formulation properties and conditions are mostly unknown and a large formulation design space needs to be investigated, the miniaturized, high-throughput LOC technologies provide a valuable alternative to traditional techniques because of the low requirements for sample amounts, high flexibility of sample preparation, and capability to screen a large variety of formulations in a very short time.

A list of analytical methods that are suitable for high-throughput and/or automated analysis of protein formulations during the preclinical and clinical development stages is provided in Table 3.1. Many of these methods listed in Table 3.1 have been also discussed in the previous Chapters 1 and 2. The focus of preclinical formulation development is the selection of a formulation for a lead candidate that is suitable for First-in-Human and Phase 1 clinical studies. At this point of development it is common that the number of formulations that need to be screened is fairly large, as are the number of characterization assays.

3.2 Modality-specific formulation screening

Formulation development can be platform-based with well-defined studies and methods for formulation screening and characterization that are specific to a structural template of a therapeutic agent (i.e., modality). However, platform-based development needs time to mature to a point where a molecular modality is well characterized and

Table 3.1 **High-throughput methods for formulation characterization that can be used for biopharmaceutical pre-clinical formulation development**

Quality attribute	Method	Characteristics	References
Conformational stability	Freeze–thaw cycling	Aggregation	[14]
	Differential static light scattering (DSLS)	Aggregation	[15]
	Differential scanning fluorimetry (DSF)	Unfolding, aggregation	[16–19,21,32]
	Fluorescence spectroscopy	Aggregation, interface interaction	[19,33]
	UV spectroscopy	Conformation, aggregation	[34]
	Temperature-ramped turbidity	Unfolding, aggregation	[35]
	Small-angle X-ray scattering	Structure	[36]
Colloidal stability	Differential static light scattering (DSLS)	Aggregation	[15]
	Differential scanning flourimetry (DSF)	Aggregation	[21,37–40]
	Self-interaction nanoparticle spectroscopy	k_D, aggregation, G_{22}	[23]
	Static light scattering (SLS)	Aggregation, large particle formation	[38]
	Asymmetrical flow field-flow fractionation (AF4)	Large particle formation	[37]
	Ammonium sulfate precipitation	Solubility, aggregation propensity	[41]
Chemical modifications	Analytical ion-exchange chromatography	Charge variants	[21]
	Analytical reversed-phase chromatography	Cleavage products/ fragments	[20]

understood. Only then studies and methods can be deployed that are universally applicable and not candidate or product specific. With new emerging modalities moving into biopharmaceutical pipelines and the structural diversity of biotherapeutic candidates growing, it is critical for platform development to generate data sets that comprehensively describe the structural properties and solution behavior of a molecule class to gain access to the efficiencies and cost savings that are inherent to platform development as quickly as possible. To this end, the initial approaches to formulation development should be tailored to the structural properties and solution behavior specifically to a modality. For example, the formulation development of a peptide-based drug candidate requires formulation study designs that are quite different from studies for the development of full length protein therapeutic. Vaccine formulations, in particular, are very different from protein formulations in terms of their stability profile sensitivity of temperature, formulation excipients (e.g., surfactants), and pH. One of the most common modalities in drug development today are mAbs, typically of the IgG1 or IgG2 type. More recently, this antibody-based modality is undergoing significant diversification. In some cases, only small structural changes are introduced, in other cases more dramatic changes or additions are made to the original antibody structures with new structural properties and solution behaviors. For example, the formulations that are providing stability for mAbs are not necessarily sufficient to stabilize antibody–drug conjugates (ADCs) [42] or bispecific antibody modalities [43]. High-throughput methodologies are particularly helpful for accelerating the development and execution of both formulation screening studies and analytical methods. The resulting data sets are generally comprehensive enough to identify a formulation design space that is appropriately suited for a formulation that is sufficiently stable for Phase 1 and Phase 2 clinical studies. Due to the high-throughput format, a larger number of formulations, storage, and degradation-inducing stress conditions can be screened in much shorter periods of time and with much less material than with traditional study designs and analytical methodologies. This allows formulation scientists to expand the investigation of the initial formulation space and to generate a more complete understanding of a drug candidate's physicochemical properties. In the long term, repeating these type of high-throughput analyses with different drug candidates of the same structural template, will provide the data sets to develop platform processes that can be applied universally to a class of therapeutic agents (i.e., modality).

As mentioned above, the number of biotherapeutic modalities is growing, and in addition to current structural templates like fusion proteins, ADCs, as well as bi- and multispecific molecules, more complex molecular constructs are entering various stages of drug development. Antibody-targeted lipidic nanotherapeutics [44], antibody-decorated polymeric filomicelles [45], and functionalized carbon nanotubes [37] are just a few examples of the growing number of biotherapeutic modalities. A commendable review on formulation technology applied to colloidal nanocarriers was published by Mishra et al. [38]. For new modalities, formulation development should be focused on the physicochemical properties of individual structural components of the construct, as well as the entire construct. Additionally, the specific interactions between the individual structural components need to be investigated and understood because they may result in unique stability properties and behaviors in solution as a function of excipients and pH. In ADCs the addition of a hydrophobic cytotoxic agent to the interchain sulfhydryl groups of the antibody generates a very heterogeneous distribution of drug load. Monomethyl auristatin E (MMAE) attached to mAb molecules significantly increases the aggregation propensity in formulations with high ionic strengths and it also decreases the conformational stability of ADCs [46]. For some modalities the formulation properties are critical for the activity of the active ingredient in vivo. Lipid-based and polymer-based carrier systems containing siRNA were investigated for their hemocompatibility by Yousefi et al. [33]. It was found that the polymer-based formulation induced high platelet activation in in vitro assays, while the lipid-based formulation was less active in the activation and aggregation of platelets. Experiments like these serve as good examples for high-throughput in vitro formulation studies that can significantly reduce the number of required animal studies to predict efficacy, specificity, and safety in vivo.

Vaccines such as the virus-like particle (VLP) are another modality of biopharmaceutical drugs that require a specialized approach for formulation development. The main concern of VLP formulations is its high tendency to aggregate. Multidimensional stability data are highly desirable in early formulation development stages of VLP vaccines. Limited amounts of VLP material at this stage make it difficult to screen large numbers of formulations and conditions. Miniaturized high-throughput methodologies have been developed to study the aggregation propensity of a VLP vaccine [34]. The methodology combines dynamic light scattering (DLS) with asymmetrical flow field-flow fractionation (AF4). A DLS plate reader was used to prescreen a large formulation space to select a smaller set of formulations and conditions for further testing by flow fractionation at higher resolution. The DSL method requires only 2 μg of sample and takes about 1–2 minutes per measurement. Commonly used excipients such as polysorbate 20, sucrose, trehalose, mannitol, and sorbitol were screened at elevated temperature. The results showed that mixtures of polysorbate and sucrose stabilize the VLP vaccine during exposure to elevated temperatures and also increase the recovery of activity after freeze-drying. Another example is the formulation development of a VLP vaccine against the Chikungunya virus during which the vaccine was characterized and screened for optimal solubility and stability [47]. Generally recognized as safe, excipients were screened using a high-throughput turbidity-based assay. The concentrations and combinations of excipients were optimized and the effect of polyanions on the aggregation propensity of the vaccine was evaluated. Various strategies for stable vaccine formulations are described in the review by Kumru et al. [48]. Vaccine modalities include live, attenuated, and inactivated forms, as well as recombinant proteins. Different high-throughput methodologies have been used to screen for the best vaccine stabilizers. To evaluate the effect of excipients on antigen aggregation at air–liquid interfaces, a high-throughput method was developed that is compatible with low protein concentrations [32]. Microplates, containing various excipients, were exposed to air bubbling to induce protein aggregation. Tryptophan fluorescence measured by a fluorescence plate reader was used to evaluate the antigen's aggregation propensity. SE-HPLC, turbidimetry, Nile Red fluorescence spectroscopy, and attenuated total reflection Fourier-transform infrared spectroscopy were also used to quantify antigen aggregation. The results demonstrated that the aggregation profile determined by the high-throughput method was comparable with the profile obtained by other low-throughput techniques. Of the 44 excipients, 7 significantly decreased the aggregation propensity of the antigen at the air–liquid interface. In many cases, a simple, single assay can be as effective as an array of multiple methods. Ultraviolet absorption spectroscopy has been utilized to develop a high-throughput screening methods for measuring the conformational stability of recombinant antigenic proteins in the presence of the same 44 excipients described above [49]. Microplate-based UV spectroscopy data were analyzed by applying second-derivative transformation and compared with the data obtained by tryptophan fluorescence spectroscopy and DSF. The second-derivative

UV spectroscopy data showed that the screening resolution was comparable with that of the tryptophan fluorescence spectroscopy and DSF assays. Adjuvants are essential and serve as critical components in vaccine formulations. They are supposed to stimulate an immunogenic response and act alone, as well as in a synergetic manner, to amplify the response. A multiplexed high-throughput nanoimmunoassay chip has been introduced for screening large numbers of vaccine formulations, containing up to 10 different adjuvants and their combinations [50]. A total of 435 conditions were tested for synergetic production of inflammatory cytokines from dendritic cells. In vivo experiments confirmed the selection of the best adjuvants by the chip-based method. This matrix-insensitive and low-volume, high-throughput technology can accelerate the development of vaccine formulations at very early stages of vaccine development. DSF can be applied not only to the screening of protein stability in solution but also to vaccine formulation development [51]. The exposure of hydrophobic side chains during virus uncoating increases the fluorescence of extrinsic probes and can be used as an indication of capsid protein unfolding and overall vaccine formulation stability. The early phases of vaccine formulation development include forced degradation studies to obtain information about possible degradations and degradation pathways, to support analytical method development and to identify optimal vaccine formulations for short- and long-term storage [52].

The diversity of formulations is not limited by the variety of modalities. In addition to liquid, frozen, or lyophilized formulation types, other formulation types, depending on the indication, route of administration, and delivery system should be considered for development. The ability of certain biopharmaceutical products to crystallize may be both advantageous and detrimental for formulation development. On one hand, crystallized protein formulations can deliver stable protein formulations at very high protein concentrations. On the other hand, the formation of crystals in liquid or lyophilized formulations can prevent efficient delivery of drug product and it may induce additional degradations because of changes in pH and surface interaction at crystal–liquid or crystal–solid phase interfaces. To aid the selection of formulations with either the highest or least probability to crystallize, an automated, high-throughput centrifuge-based microfluidic system was developed [53], which represents a nice example of high-throughput screening technologies for optimizing crystalline protein formulations.

In the development of ADCs, site-specific conjugation can dramatically improve overall stability and efficacy. Due to the inherent heterogeneity of ADCs, traditional methods for conjugation site identification such as peptide mapping-based techniques are producing very complicated chromatographic profiles that are difficult to interpret. Alternatively, rapid analysis of ADCs with the help of matrix-assisted laser desorption/ionization time-of-flight mass spectrometry (MALDI-TOF) coupled with immunoaffinity capture [54] can be used for the characterization of bioconjugation sites. Two relatively novel assays were used for this method; i.e., surface-enhanced laser dissociation/ionization (SELDI) and mass spectrometry immunoassay (MSIA). The conjugated peptides were captured by an immobilized antibody targeted against the "warhead" portion of the conjugated antibody. Additionally, the mapping of conjugation sites was also used to characterize the distribution profiles of the azetidinone and *N*-hydroxysuccinimide linkers.

One of the most promising approaches in cancer therapy is the use of nanocarriers, which provide highly specific recognition of a target and rapid internalization of the toxic load to reduce systemic toxicity and increase cytotoxicity to cancer cells. An example of such a nanocarrier system has been recently described by Hapuarachchige et al. [55]. In their work a two-component delivery product was designed using an ant-HER2 humanized mAb conjugated with azide groups. The drug component was dibenzylcyclooctyne (DBCO) substituted albumin linked to paclitaxel. These components create cross-linked clusters of HER2 receptors, modified antibody, and paclitaxel-loaded nanocarriers on the cell surface. As a result of clustering, significant internalization of the complex and significant cytotoxicity in HER2-positive BT-474 breast cancer cells occurs.

The increasing diversity of biologic modalities forces formulation development also to diversify and become more complex. A wide formulation space and multidimensional characterization is required to find the optimal conditions for stable storage and delivery. High-throughput screening technologies are able to aid both the analysis of a large number of samples and application of comprehensive sets of analytical methods for the generation of quantitative parameters of product quality attributes. High flexibility and integrability make it easy to apply high-throughput systems to preclinical formulation development of many types of biopharmaceutical products, including well characterized molecules, development of which use universal platform approaches and very complex modalities, which can include proteins, viruses, and non-organic materials.

3.3 How to predict long-term stability of formulations

The structural complexity of biopharmaceutical products and the multitude of possible degradation pathways make it difficult to predict stability over a long period of time. A formulation has to be robust enough to maintain a drug's activity and efficacy, as well as its safety for patients over storage periods of 1–2 years. The preference toward the development of liquid formulations, which from a patient perspective can be more conveniently administered and are easier to produce and manageable from a supply chain perspective than for example lyophilized drug product formulations, dictates tighter specifications for formulation development. The highly competitive environment of the biopharmaceutical industry creates increasing pressure on producing commercial biotherapeutics with longer shelf-life stability faster and more efficiently. The ability to develop the capability to predict stability of drug candidates during the phase of preclinical development has the potential to significantly accelerate the development and optimization of drug product formulations during commercial and later stage development. A lot of development time can be saved by moving away from empirical experimentation to verification studies that confirm the stability predictions.

Protein degradation can follow a number of different pathways depending on the production, handling, and storage conditions. Usually chemical degradations are better understood, easier to predict, and are therefore better controllable. Traditionally, the recommended storage temperature of liquid parenterals is 2–8°C. Additional challenges arise from an increasing demand for formulations to be stable at ambient and even higher temperatures. Storage at elevated temperatures not only increases the kinetic rates for chemical reactions but also the propensity of physical degradations such as protein aggregation and particulation. The formation of small soluble aggregates, as well as larger subvisible and visible protein particles, has been a focus of the regulatory agencies because of the possibility of unwanted immunological reactions, loss of efficacy, or other adverse effects [56]. A common approach to test the stability of proteins in solution is to store relatively large numbers of samples at predetermined conditions for a long period of time, normally 1–3 years. Typically, and particularly during commercial formulation development, the use of sample volumes and product containers that represent the commercial drug product configuration, such as 5 cc glass vials or 1–2 mL prefilled syringes is required. These costly and lengthy studies involve a large amount of material and many hours of manual labor. In some cases, depending on the study design and conditions selected to evaluate long-term stability, the results are not always predicting commercial product stability very well. Currently, there is a call for study designs and analytical assays that allow the development of models that predict long-term stability more accurately to eliminate the need for laborious, lengthy, and not always appropriately stability indicating studies. As mentioned before, it would be ideal to base stability predicting models on structure-based calculations. However, the understanding of the relationship between structural properties and aggregation propensity is still too limited in the academic and industry community to allow the development of computational algorithms that predict a protein's stability, solubility, or propensity to aggregate accurately and reliably. On the other hand, experimental methods to evaluate protein aggregation have been applied in biopharmaceutical development for a long time. Conformational stability is among the most common characteristics to be tested. Aforementioned DSF and several other assays are very well suited to screen protein formulations for conformational stability in a high-throughput format [25,57–60]. Temperature-induced unfolding is widely used to predict long-term protein stability. A good correlation between the melting temperature T_m and aggregation propensity during incubation at 40°C has been observed for mAbs [16]. This correlation seems to make sense because it implies that the closer a protein's unfolding temperature is to the incubation temperature the higher the probability the protein starts to unfold and upon the loss of its native structure to aggregate. The problem with studies that use the mechanism of temperature-induced aggregation to predict long-term stability is that they do not necessarily predict well long-term stability at low temperatures. Since most proteins are conformationally stable at temperatures between 2°C and 8°C, the mechanism of aggregation at low temperatures is based on native self-association (colloidal stability) rather than on non-native protein–protein interactions (conformational stability). Even though significant progress has been made over the last 5 years, the prediction of long-term stability is still lacking reliable methodologies [61]. Whether the mechanism of protein aggregation is based on native or non-native protein–protein interactions is depending on the particular formulation properties and storage conditions. Measuring the rate of aggregation at elevated temperatures is an approach to study protein–protein interactions as a function of non-native conformational properties at a point when the protein is starting to unfold and non-native structural conformations expose residues and surfaces that are prone to self-association. The rate-limiting step of high temperature-induced aggregation can be fitted by appropriate models to predict the aggregation propensity at lower temperatures [62,63]. One method to measure the initial rate of protein aggregation is to incubate protein samples at elevated temperatures and analyze aliquots of these samples by size-exclusion ultra high-performance liquid chromatography (SE-UHPLC) after defined periods of time. Modern SE-UHPLC assays use multi-well plates, usually 96-well plates, and ultra high-pressure columns that operate at up to 20,000 psi. As a result analysis times can be decreased down to a few minutes. Assuming that aggregation at low temperatures is caused by self-association of native monomeric proteins, protein–protein interactions between structurally stable proteins should be used as the underlying mechanism for the development of stability predicting models. The tendency of natively folded and stable proteins to remain dispersed in solution and not to self-associate is also called colloidal stability and was mentioned in Chapter 2; Early stage formulation development and candidate selection. There, high-throughput solubility screens were used to select the candidates with the highest colloidal stability, or in other words those candidates that had the lowest tendency to self-associate as a function of increasing protein concentrations. Banks et al. [41] applied the principle of colloidal stability to correlate protein solubility in solutions with different concentrations of ammonium sulfate with long-term stability of mAbs as a function of protein concentration and excipient type. To this end, the aggregation data, obtained after more than 1 year of storage at 4°C and 25°C, were correlated with the ammonium sulfate concentration necessary to precipitate the protein in the presence of different excipients. In Fig. 3.1 the concentration of protein left in solution after precipitation by ammonium sulfate is plotted against the concentration of ammonium sulfate in solution. The data plotted include formulations with different excipients, which correspond to different labels. The two panels present precipitation data generated at two temperatures; i.e., 4°C and 25°C. The correlation between percentage of aggregates measured by SE-HPLC and the amount of protein that remained soluble following precipitation at a given concentration of ammonium sulfate is shown in the inserts for different mAbs. In addition to the experimental measurements, the native-state transfer free energy was used as a determinate of protein solubility and colloidal stability. The degree of interaction of each of the excipients with the native mAb was estimated on the basis of the free transfer energy of an amino acid from water into an excipient solution (ΔG_{tr}), which is equal to the difference in the standard-state chemical potentials according to

$$\Delta G_{tr} = \Delta\mu^\circ = RT\ln\left(\frac{S_w}{S_e}\right) + RT\ln\left(\frac{\gamma_w}{\gamma_e}\right), \tag{3.1}$$

where S is the molar concentration of the amino acid at its solubility limit in water (S_w) and excipient (S_e), and γ_w and γ_e are the corresponding activity coefficients. The calculated ΔG_{tr} values are "apparent" ΔG_{tr} values, and such values for amino acids and model units of the peptide backbone have been previously determined in the presence of several excipients and described elsewhere [64,65]. Assuming that the

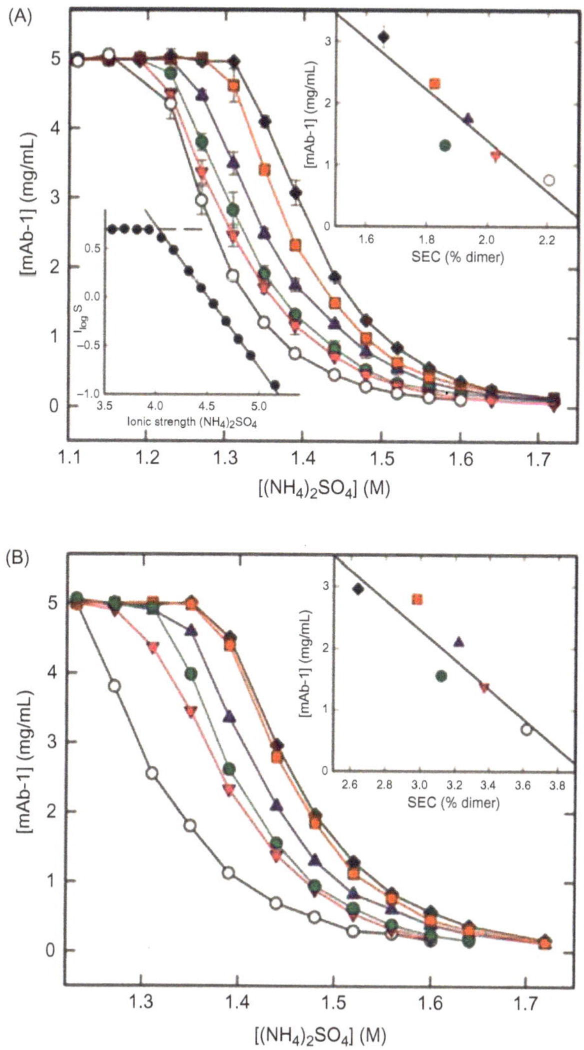

Figure 3.1 Ammonium sulfate precipitation of 5 mg/mL mAb-1 buffered at pH 5.2 with 10 mM sodium acetate conducted at 4°C (A) and 29°C (B) in the presence of 270 mM of the following excipients: sucrose (■), sorbitol (●), glycerol (▲), L-proline (◆), in the absence of excipient (▼), and in the presence of 2% (w/v) PEG-6000 (○). The amount of mAb-1 that remained soluble following precipitation at a given concentration of ammonium sulfate correlated well with the amount of dimer generated after 11.25 and 5.75 months of storage at 4°C and 29°C, respectively, in the same solvent conditions used for the precipitation experiments (minus the ammonium sulfate). Representative correlations to the amount of mAb-1 that remained soluble following ammonium sulfate precipitation at 1.39 and 1.42 M for 4°C and 29°C are shown in the upper insets of Panel (A) and Panel (B), respectively. Essentially, the amount of mAb-1 that remained soluble following precipitation could be determined at any concentration of ammonium sulfate by fitting the log of the mAb-1 concentration; a representative fit for the L-proline data is shown in the lower inset of Panel (A). *Source*: From D.D. Banks, R.F. Latypov, R.R. Ketchem, J. Woodard, J.L. Scavezze, C.C. Siska, et al., Native-state solubility and transfer free energy as predictive tools for selecting excipients to include in protein formulation development studies, J. Pharm. Sci. 101 (8) (2012) 2720–2732, Figure 6.

apparent ΔG_{tr} of all exposed groups of the folded protein are additive, the apparent $\Delta G_{tr,N}$ from water to excipient is determined using them together:

$$\Delta G_{tr,N} = \sum n_i \alpha_i \Delta g_i, \tag{3.2}$$

where n_i is the number of an amino acid or backbone unit i of the protein, Δg_i is the apparent transfer free energy for the side chain of amino acid i (or peptide backbone unit), and α_i is the fraction of surface area of the amino acid side chain or backbone unit i exposed to solvent in the native state, determined from the protein's three-dimensional structure or model. In this study the authors tried to establish a correlation between the apparent transfer free energy of the native state ($\Delta G_{tr,N}$) and the native-state solubility of three antibodies, incubated at 4°C. The results indicated that the stabilizing effect of excipients formulated at isotonic concentrations is derived from their ability to solubilize the native state, not by the increase of protein conformational stability induced by their presence. The most stabilizing excipient was proline and the least stabilizing was glycerol. However, it is possible that the rank order of excipients change. If a protein had a greater ratio of Asn and Gln to Asp and Glu residues, it may be expected that it would aggregate to a lesser extent in sucrose than proline on the basis of these side-chains ΔG_{tr} values into both excipients. This study also indicated that at low temperatures, no apparent correlation between conformational stability measured by DSC and aggregation exists. Solubility predictions based on calculating the transfer free energy is as or even more accurate than the more time consuming solubility measurements by protein precipitation. The only caveat of using such calculation is that it requires the three-dimensional structure of the protein, which could be difficult to acquire in cases when a protein is difficult to crystallize or too large for NMR. Higher concentrations of ammonium sulfate are needed to precipitate antibodies in formulations that contain a solubility increasing excipient. At 4°C, after incubation for 1–2 years, the amount of aggregates, which were mostly comprised of dimeric antibody molecules, was less than 5%. The accuracy of these solubility measurements depends on how the protein concentration was determined after precipitation. In theory, precipitation concentration of ammonium sulfate is not dependent on protein concentration, but the effect of macromolecular crowding can interfere with salt-induced self-association mechanism at concentrations where the distance between molecules is comparable with their size. Direct absorption measurements at 280 nm have absorption limits for maintaining a linear response between absorption and protein concentration. Alternatively, automated SE-HPLC can be used to estimate the protein concentration by calculating the chromatographic peak area. The sensitivity of the measurement is depended on the column properties and the dimensions of the detector flow cell. After ammonium sulfate addition, samples have to be mixed thoroughly by pipetting or mechanical shaking, and incubated for more than 3 hours to establish an equilibrium between the precipitate and solution phase. Following incubation, samples are centrifuged at their incubation temperature. The supernatants are diluted with water or they are transferred directly for protein concentration measurements. If a plate reader is used, additional care should be taken to properly seal the plate wells to stop solvent from evaporating, which may lead to inaccurate results.

Although these types of studies contribute to an increasing understanding of the relationship between native-state solubility and non-native aggregation, there is still a lot to be learned. For instance, in some cases conformational and colloidal stability may play interchangeable or equally important roles in the mechanism of protein stability. In a recent study by Banks et al., native-state solubility and non-native aggregation of recombinant human granulocyte colony stimulating factor (rhGCSF) was investigated [66]. At the recommended formulation storage temperature at 2–8°C, rhGCSF is stable with a low propensity to aggregate. At physiological temperatures and at neutral pH, the secondary structure of rhGCSF is significantly altered and forms irreversible and covalently cross-linked aggregates because of the presence of a free cysteine thiol at position 17 [67]. In the study by Banks et al., strong correlations were found between rhGCSF non-native aggregation and both solubility and thermal stability as a function of sucrose concentration. Solubility was quantified by measuring the protein concentration after incubation at different temperatures or different sucrose and potassium phosphate concentrations. In Fig. 3.2A the rhGCSF solubility dependence on temperature and sucrose concentration is shown. Protein solubility usually decreases with decreasing temperature. In the case of rhGCSF, however, the opposite is observed. The solubility in the presence of potassium phosphate rapidly decreases below 0.2 M potassium phosphate and follows the same inverse temperature dependence (Fig. 3.2B). The advantage of this phenomenon is that the solubility of this particular protein can be measured at more physiologically relevant ionic strengths, which gives this method an advantage over other methods that are depending on extrapolations from solubility curves obtained by ammonium sulfate or PEGs precipitation. The solubility surface for sucrose shown in Fig. 3.2A was fitted by the exponential function

$$f(X,T) = b\exp(m_x X + m_T T), \tag{3.3}$$

where X and T represent the sucrose concentration and temperature, respectively; m are the exponential constants and b is the common intercept. The temperature solubility surface for potassium phosphate (Fig. 3.2B) has been fitted by two exponential curves $f(X, T)$, similar to sucrose solubility, with the exception that potassium phosphate solubility is equal to

$$[(f(X,T)_{\text{salt-in}})^{-1} + (f(X,T)_{\text{salt-out}})^{-1}]^{-1}. \tag{3.4}$$

rhGCSF aggregation was induced by incubation at 37°C at concentrations below the solubility limit. SE-HPLC analysis determined the amount of soluble protein left in solution after incubation. The half-time, or the time required for half of the initial concentration of protein to be lost to insoluble aggregates, was determined by fitting the integrated peak area of the SE-HPLC chromatogram as a function of time to a sigmoidal equation explaining a nucleation mechanism [68], which seems adequate to describe

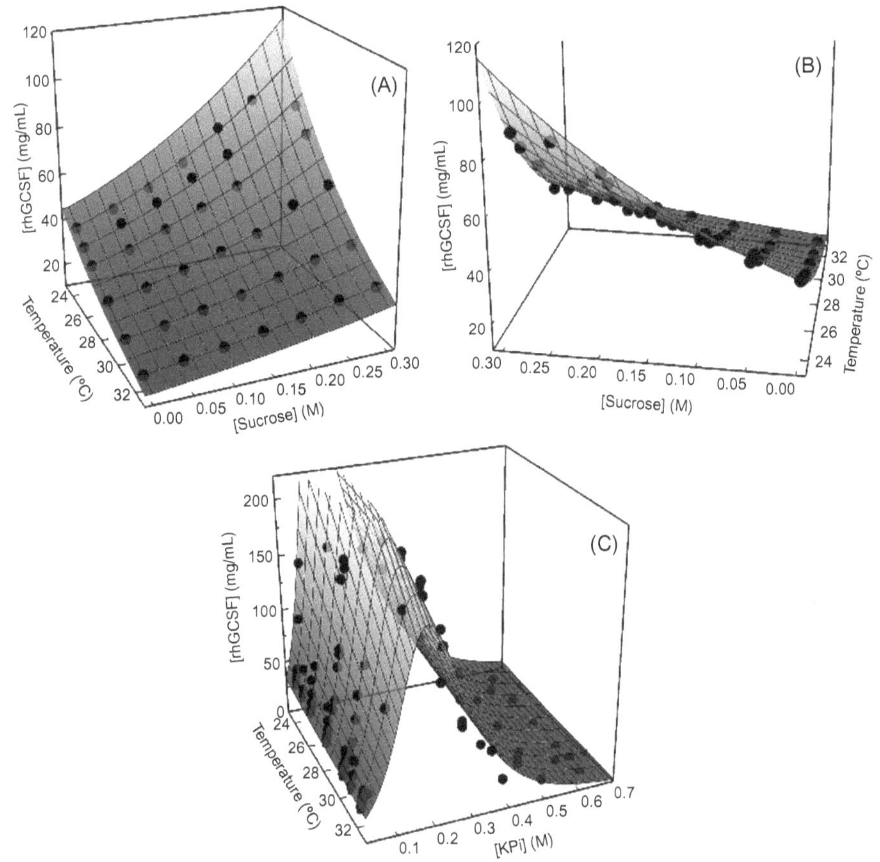

Figure 3.2 (A) rhGCSF solubility dependence on temperature and sucrose concentration (buffered with 30 mM KPi, pH 7.1). These data are also shown rotated horizontally (B) to highlight the slight twist in the surface. (C) rhGCSF temperature–KPi (pH 7.1) concentration solubility surface. Data (●) were fit globally (gray surfaces) to a single (A and B) or sum of two (C) exponential equations of the type shown in the equation in the text (Eq. 3.3), incorporating the equation of a line for *mX* and *mT* as described.
Source: From D.D. Banks, J. Zhang, C.C. Siska, Relationship between native-state solubility and non-native aggregation of recombinant human granulocyte colony stimulating factor: practical implications for protein therapeutic development, Mol. Pharm. 11 (10) (2014), 3431–3442, Figure 2.

rhGCSF aggregation according to previously published data [69]. Based on these results and the data of the temperature dependence of urea-induced unfolding experiments, a new interpretation of the early steps of aggregation was proposed to explain the native-state solubility and aggregation correlation. The proposed mechanism of aggregation includes the existence of a native monomer preequilibrium state, which is highly dependent on temperature and contains well-populated intermediate species of greater solvent exposure. The presence of native and intermediate species is consistent with the work by Roberts et al., where the equilibrium is established much faster than the aggregation processes [70]. Association between monomers is usually rate limiting and the rate of soluble monomer loss is dependent on the concentration of an intermediate state monomer. The addition of excipients that interact unfavorably with the protein surface of the native state can enrich the population of more compact, less solvent-exposed species and can prevent dimer formation, which is the initial step in the aggregation process. To this end, the measurement of the proportion of the rhGCSF intermediate state monomer should be predictive of the aggregation rate. The high-throughput method of solubility screening described in the study can be used to generate data that can be used to predict the aggregation propensity of proteins as a function of formulation composition and pH. The methods for solubility screening do not require sophisticated methodologies and instruments like other methods to measure colloidal stability. Concentration measurements are sufficiently adequate to accurately quantify the level of solubility during specified incubation conditions. Interestingly, the results of this study were able to demonstrate that solubility screening can also be applied to conditions that induce protein aggregation through non-native protein–protein interactions. However, the presence of unfolded protein in solution may complicate the measurements and additional control experiments are commonly required. The methodology may not work if the aggregation rate is limited by unfolding rather than self-association. Another problem is related to the fact that different excipients and conditions may affect the equilibrium between the native and intermediate states.

Other precipitating agents that have been used for solubility measurements and quantitative evaluation of colloidal stability are differently sized polyethylene glycols (PEGs). The effect of PEG molecules on solubility, stability, and conformation was studied and shown to be dependent on the size of the PEG polymer as subtle changes in protein conformation can significantly affect a protein's propensity to precipitate [71]. PEG-induced precipitation conducted in a high-throughput format has been successfully applied to screen the solubility of IgG1 mAbs [72], and it is just a matter of time when it will be applied more broadly to a wide variety of different precipitation assays to screen solubility during biopharmaceutical formulation development.

One form of colloidal instability is liquid–liquid phase separation (LLPS), which can be induced by PEG and has been used to evaluate quantitative parameters of antibody solutions [73]. The theory of LLPS has been developed in the area of colloidal chemistry and the phenomenon of LLPS is well established and studied for spherical colloidal particles [74]. Typically, LLPS of mAb solutions occurs only under conditions with a rare combination of temperature, protein concentration, and specific properties of the protein molecule. At temperatures above the freezing point of the solution, intermolecular interactions of antibody molecules are often too weak to result in LLPS. In the study by Wang et al. [73], LLPS was induced by the presence of PEG. The solubility of the studied antibodies was determined at the equilibrium concentration of the antibody in solution that is reached after incubation with different amounts of PEG at a specified temperature. It is worthwhile to point out that antibody solubility was measured at relatively low protein concentrations (1 mg/mL and below), which is beneficial for screening colloidal stability and predicting the propensity of self-association at early stages of drug development when material can be limited. To direct measurements of solubility by PEG-induced precipitation, the thermodynamic parameters of the equilibrium between liquid phases or between solution and precipitate can be used to characterize colloidal stability of antibody formulations. Solubility data obtained by precipitation or LLPS are described by an analytical equation with two major parameters: first, the difference between the volume excluded by PEG in the dilute phase and in the condensed phase $\Delta\nu$; second, the binding energy of an antibody molecule in the condensed phase ε_B, which is a characteristic of the net attractive interactions in the condensed phase. Even though ε_B is the lower estimate of the binding energy between proteins in a solid precipitate and crystal form, it is a useful parameter to consider for screening colloidal stability, and a possible predictor of long-term storage stability in cases when protein solubility is based on native protein–protein interactions of properly folded proteins. To this end, high-throughput screening studies of solubility parameters and thermodynamic values, derived from those parameters, are useful for the selection of formulations with optimal solubility and stability properties.

Another approach for predicting colloidal stability is the propensity estimation of protein self-association at low protein concentrations and conditions with no apparent evidence of aggregation. In this approach the parameter of self-association, the osmotic second virial coefficient, B_{22}, can be determined as the level of attractiveness between two protein molecules, which can be measured by a number of different methods such as self-interaction chromatography (SIC), static light scattering (SLS), and analytical ultracentrifugation (AUC) [75]. Generally, osmotic coefficients define the deviations from ideal solutions; i.e., when no interaction between protein molecules exist and when B_{22} is equal to zero. Positive B_{22} values indicate overall repulsive forces between proteins and, correspondently, negative B_{22} values indicate attractive forces between proteins, pointing at an increased propensity for aggregation. The above-mentioned methods for the measurement of the B_{22} are not exactly suited for high-throughput experimentation. In fact, they require carefully executed procedures and thorough data analysis. In the work by Le Brun et al., SIC was evaluated as a methodology for the measurement of the B_{22} coefficient of an IgG1 mAb in comparison to SLS measurements [76]. Fourier-transform infrared spectroscopy confirmed that the interaction of the antibody with the resin particles of the chromatography column did not induce any changes to the native three-dimensional structure. Acidic pH, low buffer and salt concentrations, as well as high concentrations of amino acids as added excipients resulted in positive B_{22} values, indicative of prevalent repulsive forces. Saito et al. demonstrated that negative B_{22} values correlate with increased viscosity of mAb formulations [77]. In addition, for formulations with negative B_{22} values the viscosity and aggregation propensity was also dependent on the amino acid sequence. Therefore, the individual surface properties of mAbs may contribute to the overall solution viscosity as well. Higher throughput for determining B_{22} values can be achieved by utilizing plate reader-based DLS measurements for measuring the diffusion coefficient at various protein concentrations. The diffusion interaction parameter, k_D, is determined based on the protein concentration dependence of the diffusion coefficient [35,39]. The k_D coefficient can replace the B_{22} in cases when only a qualitative estimation of the engaging forces between proteins is required. DLS-based methods in their current format are only applicable at protein concentrations lower than 15–20 mg/mL and higher than 1 mg/mL. About four to five data points at protein concentrations between 1 and 20 mg/mL are required to plot the values of the diffusion coefficient. A positive slope generally implies a positive k_D value and overall repulsive forces between the protein molecules, which in turn indicates a low propensity for self-association. Typically, antibody formulations return positive k_D values. Addition of salt greatly decreases k_D, which correlates with an increasing propensity to aggregate. For IgG1 mAbs, formulated in acetate buffer with a NaCl concentration of 60 mM, it has been shown that the level of agitation-induced particulation is increased 100- to 1000-fold with a k_D <7 mL/g [25]. High-throughput measurements of the diffusion interaction coefficient, k_D, by DLS have been also used for screening different sugars to enhance and optimize the stability of mAb formulations [36]. The obtained k_D values were shown to correlate with both aggregation rate constants and melting temperatures.

Another, recently introduced high-throughput methodology to study the correlation between thermal unfolding and aggregation is the evaluation of thermal stability with the help of temperature-ramped turbidity measurements [78]. This methodology uses DSF to measure the apparent melting temperature and the onset of the melting transitions of proteins such as therapeutic mAbs and its fragments. Temperature-ramped turbidity measurements were conducted to determine aggregate formation as a function of temperature. Appearance of small aggregates was monitored by temperature-ramped DLS to determine the diffusion interaction parameter, k_D. It was found that repulsive net charges at low pH increased the colloidal stability but at the same time were responsible for a decrease in conformational stability. At neutral pH and in the presence of salt, protein unfolding was followed by precipitation. Low, decreasing k_D values were indicating that protein aggregation was driven by hydrophobic interactions. In the work by Saluja et al. [40], unfolding thermodynamics were incorporated into the prediction of aggregation rates. It was demonstrated that aggregation of multi-domain proteins in liquid solutions can be approximately described by a second-order process. Furthermore, the authors found that the application of Arrhenius kinetics to stability data, generated under aggregation accelerating conditions, resulted in an underestimation of the aggregation rates under refrigerated, long-term storage. On the other hand, the use of the extended Lumry–Eyring model resulted in a more accurate estimate of aggregation rates under low-temperature conditions. Additionally, high protein concentrations can further complicate the prediction of aggregation rates because of non-ideal solution properties.

Small-angle X-ray scattering (SAXS) is another useful technology that is compatible with high-throughput screening methodologies for the fast comparison of protein stability as a function of formulation composition and storage condition. In the study by Tian et al. [79], conventional biophysical methods were applied to evaluate the structural, conformational, and colloidal stability of humanized IgG1, IgG2, and IgG4 mAbs with identical variable regions. The SAXS data obtained with the same sample set were compared with the data sets of conventional biophysical techniques. The high information content of SAXS data revealed structural differences between the antibody subclasses at various pH values. The detected variations in intermolecular repulsion at low protein concentrations were predictive of a decrease in aggregation propensity of the IgG1 antibody subclass. Likewise the contribution of excipients to the repulsion behavior was clearly noticeable. Therefore, in part due to its compatibility with high-throughput screening, SAXS may find wider applicability as an orthogonal technology for the selection of antibody candidates, verification of structurally engineered variants, and formulation development.

Subcutaneous delivery of concentrated mAb formulations is complicated by the propensity of mAbs to self-associate at elevated protein concentrations, which can lead to undesirable solution properties such as protein aggregation and abnormally high solution viscosity. Therefore, the selection of mAb candidates with low propensity to self-association early during the preclinical development phase can significantly reduce the time and resource that is required at later stages of clinical and commercial development. However, it is difficult to use conventional biophysical methods for measuring weak intermolecular interactions during the early phases of development given the large number of antibody candidates that need to be characterized, the low amount of available protein, and in some cases limited purity. Fortunately, significant progress has been made recently in adapting conventional biophysical methods, as well as developing new methods, for early identification of mAbs with low propensity to self-associate [80]. These advances should improve the selection of mAb candidates that are suitable for the requirements of delivering high concentrations of therapeutic proteins subcutaneously. At high protein concentrations, above 100 mg/mL, short-range forces start to increasingly contribute to colloidal interactions and therefore complicate stability predictions. To better address this problem, a new method has been developed by the group of Christopher Roberts at the University of Delaware, in which the osmotic second virial coefficient, B_{22}, was replaced by the protein concentration dependent protein–protein Kirkwood–Buff (KB) integrals, G_{22} [81]. G_{22} can be determined by SLS or DLS measurements, and it is more accurate for estimating the propensity to self-association at high protein concentrations. The same group developed coarse-grained models, which were used to calculate the steric contributions to the B_{22} [82]. The B_{22} values were in good agreement with values obtained from all-atom models. The coarse-grained modeling approach has the advantage that it requires shorter analysis times and lesser computational resources, which is specifically advantageous for the modeling of large multidomain proteins.

There is no single method that is capable of accurately predicting long-term formulation stability. It seems that several parameters need to be considered and measured to properly weigh the contributions of different possible degradation pathways. The characterization of conformational and colloidal stability can be evaluated for a variety of formulation compositions and stress-inducing conditions to develop a comprehensive understanding of all the possible aggregation mechanisms relevant to drug product storage conditions. High-throughput technologies are available for formulation screening, utilizing automated processes to obtain multiple parameters simultaneously from a single sample with limited amounts and sample volume. Even if a large amount of information about a molecule and formulation has been generated at the preclinical stage of development, it may not necessarily guarantee accurate predictions of the actual product stability during many months of storage. However, a comprehensive understanding of the evaluated formulation design space, should greatly reduce the risk of failing product development and production at the later stages of commercialization. The combination of experimental results from stability studies with structural information derived from both primary sequence and three-dimensional structure analyses should improve scientists' ability to correlate structural properties with the behavior of proteins in solution to better predict long-term formulation stability. Methods for enhanced calculation-based prediction of solubility may be included by utilizing computational tools borrowed from information and game theory. The concept of entropy in information theory, along with amino acid and dipeptide compositions were applied based on a different mode of pseudo amino acid composition [83]. The results confirmed that the introduction of entropy can significantly improve the performance of the classifiers in prediction models.

It seems plausible to predict that the accuracy of long term stability predictions will be improving with the development of more sensitive experimental methodologies and with the improved capabilities to collect information from multiple dimensions that characterize colloidal and conformational interactions that are driven by native and non-native conformations, as well as chemical modifications and their impact on structural integrity. Strong fundamental knowledge collected by a variety of physicochemical techniques and experiments investigating intermolecular interactions is probably the most critical factor in understanding how the structural and conformational properties of a protein render into favorable properties in formulation solutions. In addition, increasing computational power and increasingly sophisticated computing algorithms allow the development of predictive models with greater accuracy in identifying the critical parameters that properly predict protein stability. Experimental and theoretical methodologies eventually will result in accurate projections of both initial and long-term stability, enabling the development and deployment of platforms for more efficient and cost effective formulation and product development. It also seems plausible that high-throughput methodologies will play a significant role in enabling scientists to generate the data sets that are required for building models that are useful and sufficiently accurate in predicting the stability and properties of biotherapeutic drug product formulations.

References

[1] H.F. Liu, J. Ma, C. Winter, R. Bayer, Recovery and purification process development for monoclonal antibody production, MAbs 2 (5) (2010) 480–499.

[2] S. Chen, H. Lau, Y. Brodsky, G.R. Kleemann, R.F. Latypov, The use of native cation-exchange chromatography to study aggregation and phase separation of monoclonal antibodies, Protein Sci. 19 (6) (2010) 1191–1204.

[3] A. Johnston, E. Uren, D. Johnstone, J. Wu, Low pH, caprylate incubation as a second viral inactivation step in the manufacture of albumin: parametric and validation studies, Biologicals 31 (3) (2003) 213–221.

[4] A. Berg, M. Schuetz, F. Dismer, J. Hubbuch, Automated measurement of apparent protein solubility to rapidly assess complex parameter interactions, Food Bioprod. Process. 92 (2) (2014) 133–142.

[5] T. Ireland, H. Lutz, M. Siwak, G. Belton, Viral filtration of plasma-derived human IgG, Biopharm. Int. 17 (11) (2004) 38–44.
[6] S.E. Bondos, A. Bicknell, Detection and prevention of protein aggregation before, during, and after purification, Anal. Biochem. 316 (2) (2003) 223–231.
[7] International Conference on Harmonisation of Technical Requirements for Registration of Pharmaceuticals for Human Use (ICH). Stability Testing: Photostability Testing of New Drug Substances and Products Q1B (Step 4 Version). ICH Harmonized Tripartite Guidelines, 1996.
[8] Z. Wei, J. Feng, H.Y. Lin, S. Mullapudi, E. Bishop, G.I. Tous, et al., Identification of a single tryptophan residue as critical for binding activity in a humanized monoclonal antibody against respiratory syncytial virus, Anal. Chem. 79 (7) (2007) 2797–2805.
[9] B.A. Kerwin, R.L. Remmele, Protect from light: photodegradation and protein biologics, J. Pharm. Sci. 96 (6) (2007) 1468–1479.
[10] J. Fransson, A. Hagman, Oxidation of human insulin-like growth factor I in formulation studies, II. Effects of oxygen, visible light, and phosphate on methionine oxidation in aqueous solution and evaluation of possible mechanisms, Pharm. Res. 13 (10) (1996) 1476–1481.
[11] B.S. Bhatnagar, R.H. Bogner, M.J. Pikal, Protein stability during freezing: separation of stresses and mechanisms of protein stabilization, Pharm. Dev. Technol. 12 (5) (2007) 505–523.
[12] L. Van den Berg, The effect of addition of sodium and potassium chloride to the reciprocal system: KH_2PO_4-Na_2HPO_4-H_2O on pH and composition during freezing, Arch. Biochem. Biophys. 84 (1959) 305–315.
[13] J.F. Carpenter, B.S. Chang, W. Garzon-Rodriguez, T.W. Randolph, Rational design of stable lyophilized protein formulations: theory and practice, Pharm. Biotechnol. 13 (2002) 109–133.
[14] D. Murphy Piedmonte, C. Summers, A. McAuley, L. Karamujic, G. Ratnaswamy, Sorbitol crystallization can lead to protein aggregation in frozen protein formulations, Pharm. Res. 24 (1) (2007) 136–146.
[15] H. Trnka, J. Rantanen, H. Grohganz, Well-plate freeze-drying: a high throughput platform for screening of physical properties of freeze-dried formulations, Pharm. Dev. Technol. 20 (1) (2014) 65–73.
[16] D.S. Goldberg, S.M. Bishop, A.U. Shah, H.A. Sathish, Formulation development of therapeutic monoclonal antibodies using high-throughput fluorescence and static light scattering techniques: role of conformational and colloidal stability, J. Pharm. Sci. 100 (4) (2011) 1306–1315.
[17] O.K. Gasymov, B.J. Glasgow, ANS fluorescence: potential to augment the identification of the external binding sites of proteins, Biochim. Biophys. Acta 1774 (3) (2007) 403–411.
[18] S.D. Fowler, P. Greenspan, Application of Nile red, a fluorescent hydrophobic probe, for the detection of neutral lipid deposits in tissue sections: comparison with oil red O, J. Histochem. Cytochem. 33 (8) (1985) 833–836.
[19] A. Hawe, M. Sutter, W. Jiskoot, Extrinsic fluorescent dyes as tools for protein characterization, Pharm. Res. 25 (7) (2008) 1487–1499.
[20] F. He, D.H. Phan, S. Hogan, R. Bailey, G.W. Becker, L.O. Narhi, et al., Detection of IgG aggregation by a high throughput method based on extrinsic fluorescence, J. Pharm. Sci. 99 (6) (2010) 2598–2608.
[21] N. Stackhouse, A.K. Miller, S.H. Himanshu, A high-throughput UPLC method for the characterization of chemical modifications in monoclonal antibody molecules, J. Pharm. Sci. 100 (12) (2011) 5115–5125.

[22] D. Farnan, G.T. Moreno, Multiproduct high-resolution monoclonal antibody charge variant separations by pH gradient ion-exchange chromatography, Anal. Chem. 81 (21) (2009) 8846–8857.
[23] S. Molloy, R.M. Fesinmeyer, T. Martinez, D. Piedmonte-Murphy, M.E. Pelletier, M.J. Treuheit, et al., Optimized UV detection of high-concentration antibody formulations using high-throughput SE-HPLC, J. Pharm. Sci. 104 (2) (2015) 508–514.
[24] J. Jayaraman, J. Wu, M.C. Brunelle, A.M.M. Cruz, D.S. Goldberg, B. Lobo, et al., Plasmonic measurements of monoclonal antibody self-association using self-interaction nanoparticle spectroscopy, Biotechnol. Bioeng. 111 (8) (2014) 1513–1520.
[25] F. He, C.E. Woods, G.W. Becker, L.O. Narhi, V.I. Razinkov, High-throughput assessment of thermal and colloidal stability parameters for monoclonal antibody formulations, J. Pharm. Sci. 100 (12) (2011) 5126–5141.
[26] P.B. Taylor, S. Ashman, S.M. Baddeley, S.L. Bartram, C.D. Battle, B.C. Bond, et al., A standard operating procedure for assessing liquid handler performance in high-throughput screening, J. Biomol. Screen. 7 (6) (2002) 554–569.
[27] R.E. Majors, New developments in microplates for biological assays and automated sample preparation, LC GC Mag.-North Am.-Solut. Separat. Sci 22 (11) (2004) 1062–1072.
[28] American National Standards Institute ANSI SLAS 1-2004 (R2012), 10/12/2011.
[29] S.C. Terry, J.H. Jerman, J.B. Angell, A gas chromatographic air analyzer fabricated on a silicon wafer, IEEE Trans. Electron Devices 26 (12) (1980) 1880–1886.
[30] A. Manz, N. Graber, H.Á. Widmer, Miniaturized total chemical analysis systems: a novel concept for chemical sensing, Sens. Actuators B 1 (1) (1990) 244–248.
[31] H. Zhao, O. Graf, N. Milovic, X. Luan, M. Bluemel, M. Smolny, et al., Formulation development of antibodies using robotic system and high-throughput laboratory (HTL), J. Pharm. Sci. 99 (5) (2010) 2279–2294.
[32] S. Dasnoy, N. Dezutter, D. Lemoine, V. Le Bras, V. Préat, High-throughput screening of excipients intended to prevent antigen aggregation at air-liquid interface, Pharm. Res. 28 (7) (2011) 1591–1605.
[33] A. Yousefi, M. Lauwers, R. Nemes, T. van Holten, N. Babae, M. Roest, et al., Hemocompatibility assessment of two siRNA nanocarrier formulations, Pharm. Res. 31 (11) (2014) 3127–3135.
[34] J. Mohr, Y.P. Chuan, Y. Wu, L.H. Lua, A.P. Middelberg, Virus-like particle formulation optimization by miniaturized high-throughput screening, Methods 60 (3) (2013) 248–256.
[35] S. Yadav, J. Liu, S.J. Shire, D.S. Kalonia, Specific interactions in high concentration antibody solutions resulting in high viscosity, J. Pharm. Sci. 99 (3) (2010) 1152–1168.
[36] J. Rubin, A. Sharma, L. Linden, A.S. Bommarius, S.H. Behrens, Gauging colloidal and thermal stability in human IgG1–sugar solutions through diffusivity measurements, J. Phys. Chem. B 118 (11) (2014) 2803–2809.
[37] S. Prakash, M. Malhotra, W. Shao, C. Tomaro-Duchesneau, S. Abbasi, Polymeric nanohybrids and functionalized carbon nanotubes as drug delivery carriers for cancer therapy, Adv. Drug. Deliv. Rev. 63 (14) (2011) 1340–1351.
[38] B. Mishra, B.B. Patel, S. Tiwari, Colloidal nanocarriers: a review on formulation technology, types and applications toward targeted drug delivery, Nanomedicine 6 (1) (2010) 9–24.
[39] S. Yadav, T.M. Scherer, S.J. Shire, D.S. Kalonia, Use of dynamic light scattering to determine second virial coefficient in a semidilute concentration regime, Anal. Biochem. 411 (2) (2011) 292–296.
[40] A. Saluja, V. Sadineni, A. Mungikar, V. Nashine, A. Kroetsch, C. Dahlheim, et al., Significance of unfolding thermodynamics for predicting aggregation kinetics: a case

study on high concentration solutions of a multi-domain protein, Pharm. Res. 31 (6) (2014) 1575–1587.
[41] D.D. Banks, R.F. Latypov, R.R. Ketchem, J. Woodard, J.L. Scavezze, C.C. Siska, et al., Native-state solubility and transfer free energy as predictive tools for selecting excipients to include in protein formulation development studies, J. Pharm. Sci. 101 (8) (2012) 2720–2732.
[42] M. Leal, P. Sapra, S.A. Hurvitz, P. Senter, A. Wahl, M. Schutten, et al., Antibody–drug conjugates: an emerging modality for the treatment of cancer, Ann. N.Y. Acad. Sci. 1321 (1) (2014) 41–54.
[43] K.F. Sachsenmeier, N. Dimasi, Q. Huang, E. Sult, B. Bezabeh, R. Fleming, et al., The avidity hypothesis: comparing bispecific and monospecific antibodies in preclinical oncology models, Cancer Res. 73 (8) (2013). Suppl. 4635.
[44] D.B. Kirpotin, C.O. Noble, M.E. Hayes, Z. Huang, T. Kornaga, Y. Zhou, et al., Building and characterizing antibody-targeted lipidic nanotherapeutics, Methods Enzymol. 502 (2012) 139–166.
[45] V.V. Shuvaev, M.A. Ilies, E. Simone, S. Zaitsev, Y. Kim, S. Cai, et al., Endothelial targeting of antibody-decorated polymeric filomicelles, ACS Nano 5 (9) (2011) 6991–6999.
[46] Y.T. Adem, K.A. Schwarz, E. Duenas, T.W. Patapoff, W.J. Galush, O. Esue, Auristatin antibody drug conjugate physical instability and the role of drug payload, Bioconjug. Chem 25 (4) (2014) 656–664.
[47] R.M. Kramer, Y. Zeng, N. Sahni, L.A. Kueltzo, R.M. Schwartz, I.K. Srivastava, et al., Development of a stable virus-like particle vaccine formulation against Chikungunya virus and investigation of the effects of polyanions, J. Pharm. Sci. 102 (12) (2013) 4305–4314.
[48] O.S. Kumru, S.B. Joshi, D.E. Smith, C.R. Middaugh, T. Prusik, D.B. Volkin, Vaccine instability in the cold chain: mechanisms, analysis and formulation strategies, Biologicals 42 (5) (2014) 237–259.
[49] S. Dasnoy, V. Le Bras, V. Préat, D. Lemoine, High-throughput assessment of antigen conformational stability by ultraviolet absorption spectroscopy and its application to excipient screening, Biotechnol. Bioeng. 109 (2) (2012) 502–516.
[50] J.L. Garcia-Cordero, C. Nembrini, A. Stano, J.A. Hubbell, S.J. Maerkl, A high-throughput nanoimmunoassay chip applied to large-scale vaccine adjuvant screening, Integr. Biol. 5 (4) (2013) 650–658.
[51] T.S. Walter, J. Ren, T.J. Tuthill, D.J. Rowlands, D.I. Stuart, E.E. Fry, A plate-based high-throughput assay for virus stability and vaccine formulation, J. Virol. Methods 185 (1) (2012) 166–170.
[52] M. Hasija, L. Li, N. Rahman, S.F. Ausar, Forced degradation studies: an essential tool for the formulation development of vaccines, Vaccine 3 (2013) 11–33.
[53] G. Li, Q. Chen, J. Li, X. Hu, J. Zhao, A compact disk-like centrifugal microfluidic system for high-throughput nanoliter-scale protein crystallization screening, Anal. Chem. 82 (11) (2010) 4362–4369.
[54] L. Dai, R. Preston, M. Bacica, A. Kinhikar, B. Bolaños, R.E. Murphy, Development of a potential high-throughput workflow to characterize sites of bioconjugation by immuno-affinity capture coupled to MALDI-TOF mass spectrometry, Bioconjug. Chem 24 (1) (2012) 53–62.
[55] S. Hapuarachchige, W. Zhu, Y. Kato, D. Artemov, Bioorthogonal, two-component delivery systems based on antibody and drug-loaded nanocarriers for enhanced internalization of nanotherapeutics, Biomaterials 35 (7) (2014) 2346–2354.

[56] W. Wang, S.K. Singh, N. Li, M.R. Toler, K.R. King, S. Nema, Immunogenicity of protein aggregates—concerns and realities, Int. J. Pharm. 431 (1) (2012) 1–11.
[57] W.F. Weiss, T.M. Young, C.J. Roberts, Principles, approaches, and challenges for predicting protein aggregation rates and shelf life, J. Pharm. Sci. 98 (4) (2009) 1246–1277.
[58] F. He, C.E. Woods, E. Trilisky, K.M. Bower, J.R. Litowski, B.A. Kerwin, et al., Screening of monoclonal antibody formulations based on high-throughput thermostability and viscosity measurements: design of experiment and statistical analysis, J. Pharm. Sci. 100 (4) (2011) 1330–1340.
[59] A.A. Canutescu, A.A. Shelenkov, R.L. Dunbrack, A graph-theory algorithm for rapid protein side-chain prediction, Protein Sci. 12 (9) (2003) 2001–2014.
[60] H. Bajaj, V.K. Sharma, A. Badkar, D. Zeng, S. Nema, D.S. Kalonia, Protein structural conformation and not second virial coefficient relates to long-term irreversible aggregation of a monoclonal antibody and ovalbumin in solution, Pharm. Res. 23 (6) (2006) 1382–1394.
[61] E. Sahin, J.L. Jordan, M.L. Spatara, A. Naranjo, J.A. Costanzo, W.F. Weiss, et al., Computational design and biophysical characterization of aggregation-resistant point mutations for γD crystallin illustrate a balance of conformational stability and intrinsic aggregation propensity, Biochemistry 50 (5) (2011) 628–639.
[62] R.K. Brummitt, D.P. Nesta, L. Chang, S.F. Chase, T.M. Laue, C.J. Roberts, Nonnative aggregation of an IgG1 antibody in acidic conditions: Part 1. Unfolding, colloidal interactions, and formation of high-molecular-weight aggregates, J. Pharm. Sci. 100 (6) (2011) 2087–2103.
[63] V. Kayser, N. Chennamsetty, V. Voynov, B. Helk, K. Forrer, B.L. Trout, Evaluation of a non-Arrhenius model for therapeutic monoclonal antibody aggregation, J. Pharm. Sci. 100 (7) (2011) 2526–2542.
[64] M. Auton, D.W. Bolen, Predicting the energetics of osmolyte-induced protein folding/unfolding, Proc. Natl. Acad. Sci. U.S.A. 102 (42) (2005) 15065–15068.
[65] M. Auton, D.W. Bolen, J. Rösgen, Structural thermodynamics of protein preferential solvation: osmolyte solvation of proteins, aminoacids, and peptides, Proteins 73 (4) (2008) 802–813.
[66] D.D. Banks, J. Zhang, C.C. Siska, Relationship between native-state solubility and non-native aggregation of recombinant human granulocyte colony stimulating factor: practical implications for protein therapeutic development, Mol. Pharm. 11 (10) (2014) 3431–3442.
[67] S.W. Raso, J. Abel, J.M. Barnes, K.M. Maloney, G. Pipes, M.J. Treuheit, et al., Aggregation of granulocyte-colony stimulating factor in vitro involves a conformationally altered monomeric state, Protein Sci. 14 (9) (2005) 2246–2257.
[68] S.I. Cohen, M. Vendruscolo, C.M. Dobson, T.P. Knowles, Nucleated polymerisation in the presence of pre-formed seed filaments, Int. J. Mol. Sci. 12 (9) (2011) 5844–5852.
[69] E.Y. Chi, S. Krishnan, B.S. Kendrick, B.S. Chang, J.F. Carpenter, T.W. Randolph, Roles of conformational stability and colloidal stability in the aggregation of recombinant human granulocyte colony-stimulating factor, Protein Sci. 12 (5) (2003) 903–913.
[70] C.J. Roberts, R.T. Darrington, M.B. Whitley, Irreversible aggregation of recombinant bovine granulocyte-colony stimulating factor (bG-CSF) and implications for predicting protein shelf life, J. Pharm. Sci. 92 (5) (2003) 1095–1111.
[71] V. Kumar, V.K. Sharma, D.S. Kalonia, Effect of polyols on polyethylene glycol (PEG)-induced precipitation of proteins: impact on solubility, stability and conformation, Int. J. Pharm. 366 (1) (2009) 38–43.

[72] T.J. Gibson, K. Mccarty, I.J. Mcfadyen, E. Cash, P. Dalmonte, K.D. Hinds, et al., Application of a high-throughput screening procedure with PEG-induced precipitation to compare relative protein solubility during formulation development with IgG1 monoclonal antibodies, J. Pharm. Sci. 100 (3) (2011) 1009–1021.
[73] Y. Wang, R.F. Latypov, A. Lomakin, J.A. Meyer, B.A. Kerwin, S. Vunnum, et al., Quantitative evaluation of colloidal stability of antibody solutions using PEG-induced liquid–liquid phase separation, Mol. Pharm. 11 (5) (2014) 1391–1402.
[74] P.N. Pusey, W. Van Megen, Phase behaviour of concentrated suspensions of nearly hard colloidal spheres, Nature 320 (6060) (1986) 340–342.
[75] J.J. Valente, R.W. Payne, M.C. Manning, W.W. Wilson, C.S. Henry, Colloidal behavior of proteins: effects of the second virial coefficient on solubility, crystallization and aggregation of proteins in aqueous solution, Curr. Pharm. Biotechnol. 6 (6) (2005) 427–436.
[76] V. Le Brun, W. Friess, S. Bassarab, S. Mühlau, P. Garidel, A critical evaluation of self-interaction chromatography as a predictive tool for the assessment of protein–protein interactions in protein formulation development: a case study of a therapeutic monoclonal antibody, Eur. J. Pharm. Biopharm. 75 (1) (2010) 16–25.
[77] S. Saito, J. Hasegawa, N. Kobayashi, N. Kishi, S. Uchiyama, K. Fukui, Behavior of monoclonal antibodies: relation between the second virial coefficient (B 2) at low concentrations and aggregation propensity and viscosity at high concentrations, Pharm. Res. 29 (2) (2012) 397–410.
[78] T. Menzen, W. Friess, Temperature-ramped studies on the aggregation, unfolding, and interaction of a therapeutic monoclonal antibody, J. Pharm. Sci. 103 (2) (2014) 445–455.
[79] X. Tian, A.E. Langkilde, M. Thorolfsson, H.B. Rasmussen, B. Vestergaard, Small-angle X-ray scattering screening complements conventional biophysical analysis: comparative structural and biophysical analysis of monoclonal antibodies IgG1, IgG2, and IgG4, J. Pharm. Sci. 103 (6) (2014) 1701–1710.
[80] P.M. Tessier, J. Wu, C.D. Dickinson, Emerging methods for identifying monoclonal antibodies with low propensity to self-associate during the early discovery process, Expert Opin. Drug Deliv. 11 (4) (2014) 461–465.
[81] M.A. Blanco, E. Sahin, Y. Li, C.J. Roberts, Reexamining protein–protein and protein–solvent interactions from Kirkwood-Buff analysis of light scattering in multi-component solutions, J. Chem. Phys. 134 (22) (2011) 225103.
[82] A. Grünberger, P.K. Lai, M.A. Blanco, C.J. Roberts, Coarse-grained modeling of protein second osmotic virial coefficients: sterics and short-ranged attractions, J. Phys. Chem. B 117 (3) (2013) 763–770.
[83] N. Xiaohui, S. Feng, H. Xuehai, X. Jingbo, L. Nana, Predicting the protein solubility by integrating chaos games representation and entropy in information theory, Expert Syst. Appl. 41 (4) (2014) 1672–1679.

Late-stage and commercial formulation development

4

4.1 Development of a robust formulation design space

As outlined in the previous Chapter 3, in the early phases of formulation development (i.e., preclinical and clinical development (Phase I and II)) the focus of development is directed toward developing a sound understanding of the protein properties that are critical for the development of a viable formulation that can be commercialized and is marketable. The objective in developing a formulation for early clinical development is to demonstrate that the type of formulation and dosage form is suitable for the intended use. Therefore, early stage studies are designed to educate the formulation scientist about a protein's most critical properties and quality attributes, which in turn direct the formulation development to appropriate dosage forms that provide conformational stability, colloidal stability, and chemical stability, but also enable a scalable manufacturing process for commercialization. To promote a commercial formulation development approach clinical formulations should have close resemblance to a formulation that is commercially acceptable. Consequently, the knowledge and understanding developed in preclinical and clinical development studies are a fundamental prerequisite for the proper design of commercial development studies, which are intended to optimize and refine a robust formulation design space to ensure patient safety and drug efficacy. Patient safety and therapeutic efficacy are paramount, and early-stage formulation development studies need to deliver a formulation design space, relevant specifications, and control of the critical parameters affecting the pharmaceutical quality of a biotherapeutic.

High-throughput technologies and methodologies are exceptionally well suited to enable scientists to gain the required understanding of the formulation parameters that are critical for therapeutic quality and stability. Especially during the early phases of formulation development the integration of speed, sensitivity, and efficiency by automating processes (e.g., sample preparation, sample analysis), accelerating analytics (e.g., ultra high-performance liquid chromatography (UPLC, UHPLC), analytics suited for automation), and miniaturizing analytics (plate-based analytics with low material requirements and high sensitivity) allows scientists to characterize and address the mechanisms of protein instability while keeping pace with fast-track formulation development timelines. During late-stage and commercial formulation development the miniaturization to plate-based stability studies and analytics is of lesser priority because material is no longer a limiting factor and the final dosage form needs to become part of the formulation development to maximize protein stability. At the later phase of development, working toward Phase III clinical studies, stability studies need to be conducted in the relevant drug product container to enable the introduction of a relevant and representative dosage form into the Phase III patient population.

High-Throughput Formulation Development of Biopharmaceuticals. DOI: http://dx.doi.org/10.1016/B978-1-907568-63-3.00004-9

Conducting commercial formulation development with the representative container may slow down throughput and limit the number of samples that can be studied in a reasonable time frame. On the other hand, the objective at this stage of development is not so much the screening for the optimal formulation composition rather than the refinement and optimization of the formulation developed during early clinical formulation development. The focus lies on gaining understanding of the formulation design space that allows the manufacture of a therapeutic that performs as intended for the intended use. Robustness is the formulation's tolerance toward manufacturing parameter or component quality shifting while maintaining stability, resulting in reproducible manufacturing and consistent product quality.

To this end, the effect of all the components of a drug product formulation (response variables) are tested and characterized for their ability to control and protect (i.e., stabilize) the critical quality attributes (CQAs) of the therapeutic and to understand the boundaries beyond which the formulation fails to maintain product stability and quality. As defined by the ICH guidelines on Quality by Design (*ICH Q8(R2)*) [1], pharmaceutical development should be aimed at the design of a quality product and manufacturing process that consistently delivers the intended performance of the product. In other words, biopharmaceuticals are required to be produced in process conditions within the operational space constructed by process characterization with minimal risk for excursion to ensure product quality. The design space specifications and manufacturing controls are constructed based on the information and knowledge gained from pharmaceutical development studies.

4.2 Application of automation and high-throughput technologies for formulation design space development

The pursuit of a commercial formulation development approach by introducing a formulation to the clinic that is designed to be commercially acceptable provides greater alignment between the early and late-stage development phases and therefore creates a more streamlined and efficient development pathway for drug commercialization. On the other hand, depending on the therapeutic area and indication of interest, drug product requirements can become very complex. In fact, a drug product for late-stage clinical studies may require a dosage form that is more complex than it was for early clinical studies. The choice of container, such as a vial or syringe, as well as the consideration of a combination product with a need for a device (e.g., autoinjector) or a delivery system (e.g., intravenous infusion (IV) system, infusion pump) may impact and change the stability of a formulation. Surface interactions with plastics, metals, and different types of glass, reactions with extractables and leachables from these surfaces can lead to specific degradation mechanisms that are not thoroughly investigated during the formulation development for early clinical studies because the final dosage form is often not known at this point. The presence of silicone oil in syringes can be a factor in increasing the propensity of aggregation or particulation. The stability of drug product in bags of IV infusion systems can be negatively impacted by increased concentration of salt and decreased protein concentration. Another factor that is difficult to predict at early stages of formulation development is the drug product protein concentration for late-stage clinical studies. It has become more and more common, especially for the development of monoclonal antibody (mAb) therapeutics, to develop formulations at high protein concentrations, often exceeding 100 mg/mL. As speed to early phase clinical studies is important to assess safety and efficacy without over-investing in time and resources, extensive formulation development as a function of protein concentration is generally not performed until after the submission of the investigational new drug (IND) application for First-in-Human/Phase I and Phase II clinical studies.

As pointed out in Section 4.1, pharmaceutical development should be aimed at the design of a quality product and manufacturing process that consistently delivers the intended performance of the product. Therefore, commercial formulation development studies for late-stage clinical studies (Phase III) are ideally performed with the representative configuration of the drug product stock-keeping unit (SKU) (e.g., glass or plastic vial, prefilled glass or plastic syringe, a combination product comprised of a syringe and device (e.g., autoinjector, infusion pump)), and analytical assays and methods that are qualified and validated for formal stability and release testing. The analytical technologies and methods that are deployed during commercial development and robustness studies need to be suited for the detection and quantification of the degradation products that have been identified during the early phases of formulation development. The priority should lie on the quality, comparability, and relevance of the data in alignment with stability data generated by Quality Control, which makes sure that development data remain relevant in representing a product's stability profile. Therefore, qualified and validated product-specific and stability-indicating methods should be used whenever possible. On the other hand, as complexity of the dosage form and factors that need to be considered during commercial formulation development increase, the multivariate nature of studies for late-stage clinical development and registration have greater and more complex study requirements that result in larger sample sets and larger numbers of response variables than univariate (i.e., one-variable-at-a-time) studies that are more commonly conducted for early clinical Phase I and Phase II studies. As the number of samples increases, the amount of data generated from these experiments dramatically increases as well. Therefore, the utilization of high-throughput technologies and the automation of sample preparation and loading for multivariate studies at this stage of development are hugely beneficial to boost productivity and the quality of experimental execution and data by (1) reducing the probability of human error, (2) reducing analyst-to-analyst variability, (3) keeping analyst away from undesirable operating conditions, e.g., hazardous materials or injury-prone and nonergonomic operations (e.g., manual particle analysis by HIAC and visual inspections), and (4) giving analysts time back to work on projects that require intellectual contributions rather than manual and repetitive hands-on activities. In this context it is important to point out that based on statistical principles the quality of the data set is a direct function of the quantity of data. This becomes particularly important for instabilities that are characterized as a statistically low-occurrence event (e.g., drug product-related particulation) and are not a homogeneous and consistently occurring property. In those particular cases, large sample sizes are required to enable the observation of a low probability event [2], which in turn increases the amount of data.

So generally speaking, due to the increased complexity of the dosage form, drug product requirements, and factors that need to be considered during commercial formulation development to ensure a stable and marketable drug product, the use of fast high-throughput analytics becomes an essential capability to increase efficiency and to develop a more comprehensive understanding of the critical quality product attributes and process control parameters that define the formulation design space. Reaching this point largely eliminates the risk of failing robustness in properly designed robustness studies, which verify the formulation design space with the drug product configuration that resembles the final commercial drug product. Many major biopharmaceutical companies have implemented different modules of automation and high-throughput technologies to appropriately scope formulation development in alignment with drug product commercialization strategies. Usually formulation-screening studies comprised of a large number of components and wide ranges of parameters are followed by studies with a more targeted focus on formulation optimization and robustness. The purpose of high-throughput screening is to identify and characterize a formulation space as fast as possible that is enabling the commercialization of a drug product for its intended use with as little time and resource as possible. Early on, the results of formulation-screening studies help evaluate the initial robustness and to frame the areas of instability of a given formulation space. Considering comparability of plate-based high-throughput assays with commercial container-based studies, later stage formulation development would be able to leverage results from high-throughput screening studies with the more targeted and refined studies of commercial development to verify robustness in the commercial dosage form and drug product configuration. An ample understanding of the design space of a stable formulation can be promoted by consistent and comprehensive study designs that take advantage of automated study execution and high-throughput analytics workflows, which in turn enables formulation scientist to define formulation platforms for classes of molecules (i.e., modalities) within reasonable development time frames. Formulation platforms allow for faster cycling times of drug candidates to transition into clinical trials and avoid non-conformances incurred by process variations during manufacturing because of a formulation stability profile that is well characterized and understood. They grant savings in time and resources, and greater alignment end-to-end between upstream and downstream processes [3–5].

Traditionally methods for monitoring product quality and stability are not developed as a high-throughput application. However, developing higher throughput methods, in particular in the area of liquid chromatography can accelerate the analysis. With the introduction of ultra high-performance liquid chromatography (UHPLC) and ultra-performance liquid chromatography (UPLC) systems, smaller particle size resins (<2 μm) packed in normal length (150–300 mm) but smaller inner diameter (<4 mm) columns, analyses can be conducted at higher flow rates because of higher pressure tolerances of 600–1000 bar. The advantage of this type of chromatography is that analysis run times can be dramatically reduced from hours to a few minutes while achieving high-resolution separation even for the most complex mixtures without compromising the quality of the analytical data [6]. Size-exclusion high-performance liquid chromatography (SE-HPLC) methods are the most widely used methods to detect and separate protein aggregates from monomers. Traditionally these methods require run times of 30–60 minutes with a typical peak width of 10–60 seconds to achieve sufficient resolution for separating the different oligomer and aggregate species. With UHPLC or UPLC systems, much greater efficiencies can be accomplished with peak widths of 2–10 seconds, higher peak capacity, and significantly reduced run times of a few minutes [7]. Similar advantages apply to the charge-based separation of proteins by ion-exchange ultra high-performance liquid chromatography (IEX-UHPLC [8]). In addition, the resulting higher peak concentrations provide increasing sensitivity when combined with a mass spectrometer using electrospray ionization (ESI) sources. Since the sensitivity of mass spectrometers is dependent on the sample concentration infused into the mass detector (concentration-sensitive detector [9]), smaller peak volumes (i.e., higher peak concentrations) significantly improve signal intensities and sensitivity. These ultra high-performing chromatography–mass spectrometry technologies are particularly useful for peptide mapping analyses, where the determination of the degradation profile of a protein and the degradation rates of chemical modifications can be determined in minutes rather than hours [10].

Another challenge for analytical high-throughput chromatography methods (e.g., SE-HPLC) is the analysis of aggregates and other high-molecular oligomers in formulations with protein concentrations higher than 100 mg/mL. Depending on a protein's extinction coefficient, methods such as UPLC are typically difficult to perform because of the limited range of signal linearity at protein concentrations higher than 2–5 mg/mL. Although the first intent is to analyze formulations neat, at their actual protein concentration, in certain circumstances it is scientifically valid to evaluate and compare formulations after dilution prior to injection. In cases where dilution cannot be conducted because of protein concentration dependent monomer/dimer equilibria, an adjustment of the absorbance wavelength to slightly higher wavelengths (e.g., 235 nm) can facilitate neat injections and analysis of small volumes of sample at higher protein concentrations [11]. High viscosity of concentrated protein solutions is generally another significant obstacle for analytical assays. In particular for assays that depend on proper mixing or loading of sample through narrow orifices like needles and capillaries. In such cases, other assays are better suited for high-throughput analyses and are easily applied to the characterization of highly concentrated formulations. Differential scanning fluorimetry (DSF) can analyze the temperature-induced unfolding of proteins at a wide range of protein concentrations (from 0.1 to 100 mg/mL) for reliable measurement of thermostability. So is dynamic light scattering (DLS) for high-throughput viscosity measurements at high protein concentrations. High viscosity of formulations in prefilled syringes is a significant challenge because of its impact on syringeability and injectability. Factors such as the plunger-stopper break-loose force, maximum force (F_{max}), and dynamic glide force, as well as needle clogging and accuracy of dose delivery [12] become especially important for needle-syringe-formulation systems when the dosage forms are comprised of injectable emulsions, suspensions, liposomes, microemulsions, and microspheres. DLS measurements are very helpful in the evaluation of possible ways to decrease viscosity during development of formulations of combination products that are comprised of a biologic and a syringe or a biologic, syringe, and device (e.g., autoinjector).

Automation does not necessarily increase productivity by increasing throughput but by running continuously for extended periods of time, operating multiple operations sequentially or in parallel, and therefore increasing efficiency, consistency, turnaround times, and the ability to accommodate larger workloads. The use of autosamplers for ultra- and high-performance liquid chromatography (e.g., HPLC, UPLC, UHPLC), subvisible particle analysis by light obscuration (HIAC), microflow imaging (MFI), and automated visual inspection are advantageous as is the automation of sample and buffer preparation (e.g., study setup, creation of aliquots, and dilutions for analytical assays) by deploying automated and programmable robotic liquid and sample handling systems (e.g., Tecan, Leap, and Hamilton). In the case of MFI, the detection and measurements of particles are automated for visualization and imaging of particles by microscopy [13]. The imaging can be performed directly from the vials or syringes without drawing samples from primary containers. Inspection systems for the assessment of visible particles have been developed and implemented in actual fill-finish lines for pharmaceutical products [14]. A schematic of such a system is shown in Fig. 4.1 [15]. The critical element for reliable assessment of particles is the setup of illumination and camera positioning. Proper illumination improves image resolution and particle analysis algorithms. For this particular system two-dimensional light emitting diode (LED) arrays were selected to obtain high-definition

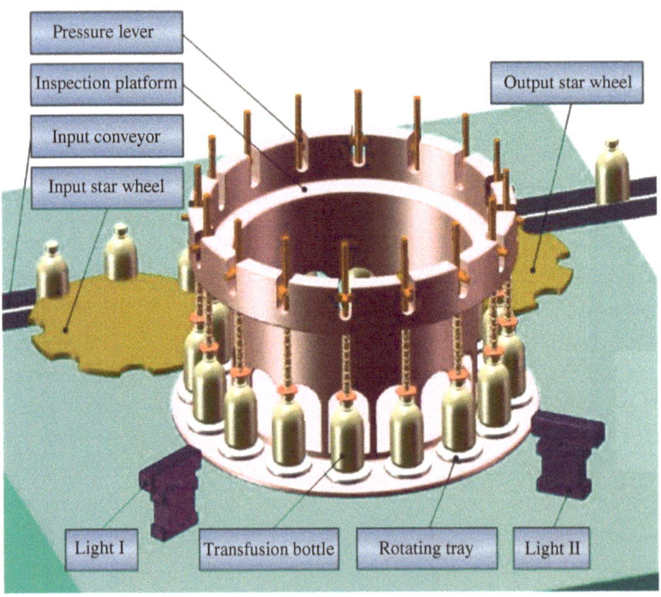

Figure 4.1 Three-dimensional drawing of an automatic inspection machine for the inspection of visible particles.

images. The containers are rotated and stopped abruptly to form a vortex that induces visible particles to move, so that they can be distinguished from cosmetic defects like scratches and other stationary spots on the surface of the container. Various software tools [16] can be applied to separate and distinguish air bubbles from the product-related particles. Discrimination of particles based on size and shape [17] along with spatial visualization of particles [18] has been successfully implemented. Automated inspection systems such as the Bausch Type 535 (Bausch Advances Technologies, Clinton, Connecticut) are employed for checking vials and syringes for embedded particles (Fig. 4.2). A robotic arm takes each vial individually from a sample tray in front of a camera system. Vials can be rotated and turned over for close-up imaging of moving particles. The sample tray holding either vials or syringes is manually inserted into the system and the containers can be accepted and returned to their original location on the tray or rejected and dropped into a reject box. The throughput is approximately several containers per minute. Automated analysis of particle counts and particle morphology is particularly useful for the classification of particles and studies investigating aggregation mechanisms.

The evaluation of freeze-dried formulations is in many aspects more complex than the analytical testing of liquid solutions. The limited understanding of excipient properties and the difficulty of analyzing product quality attributes in a solid make the characterization of freeze-dried formulations more challenging. One method to characterize a cake formed by the freeze-drying process is image analysis. Image analysis is an analytical method to obtain visual characteristics such as glassiness, the

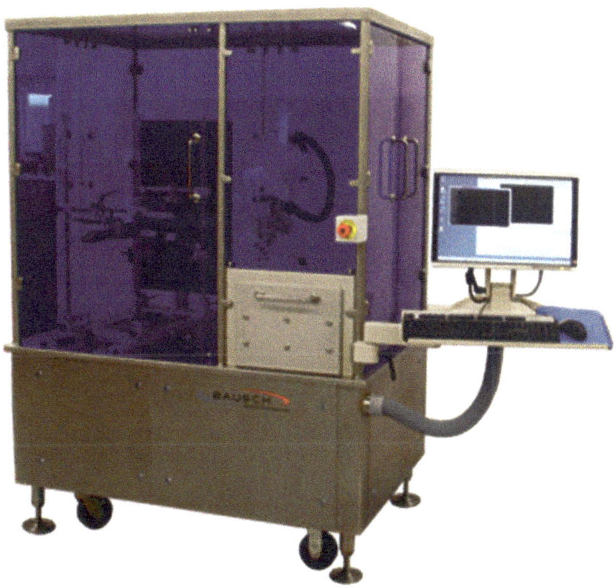

Figure 4.2 Automated syringe and vial inspection machine type 535 manufactured by Bausch.

degree of cake collapse, and color uniformity [19]. For this method, freeze-dried samples are prepared in plates. Based on the produced cake characteristics, a fuzzy logic system for analysis of this sample set of freeze-dried cakes is constructed. The system includes a measurement and learning process to recognize appropriate quality attributes of the cakes in the sample set. After this initial development phase, the system is tested with a new multi-well plate sample set. The developed fuzzy logic-based system was found to give quality scores that were comparable with the visual evaluation by human inspectors, making high-throughput classification of cake quality possible.

Another important parameter for lyophilized formulations is the time of reconstitution of freeze-dried product and product stability in the reconstituted solution. An automated method to screen and optimize the reconstitution times of multiple lyophilized formulations is described in the work by Chandran et al. [20]. Different molecules were formulated in various formulations and lyophilized in 96-well plates. The lyophilized cakes were reconstituted, and the time of complete reconstitution was measured as a function of increased transmittance within the wells over time monitored by UV absorbance with the help of a plate reader. The resulting reconstitution times obtained by plate-based measurement were in good agreement with the results obtained from conventional experiments that execute manual reconstitution. This high-throughput and miniaturized assay provides a fast and efficient way of screening for formulations with optimal reconstitution properties, and can be easily integrated into automated processes.

A key property of a freeze-dried formulation is the water (or moisture) content. Knowing and controlling the moisture content is important because it is impacting cake stability and appearance, as well as product stability. The amount of water in a freeze-dried sample is most commonly measured by Karl Fischer titration [21], which is a low-throughput method. Near infrared (NIR) spectroscopy can be used to measure moisture in freeze-dried formulations with higher throughput. The high-throughput method developed by Trnka et al. [22] is based on NIR imaging to screen freeze-dried formulation samples on multi-well plates. In this method, Karl Fischer titration was used to create the reference values and a univariate quantification model, based on NIR images, was constructed and used to visualize the distribution of water within freeze-dried samples. The results were independently confirmed by X-ray powder diffraction.

A combination of experimental design, high-throughput methods, and predictive modeling of formulation design space parameters was presented in a study investigating the formation of mannitol hemihydrate in freeze-dried protein formulations [23]. A design of experiments (DOE) study was applied to systematically investigate the impact of mannitol hemihydrate on the stability of pharmaceutical formulations by developing and leveraging response surface models. A composite face-centered design, applied in the study, used the overall solid content, protein concentration, protein type, and the ratio between mannitol and sucrose as formulation factors. Annealing was also included as a process factor in a full factorial design. For two proteins, the study resulted in models with a high goodness fit and goodness of prediction. High protein concentration, low relative mannitol content, and annealing at low temperature were the most significant factors for enhancing the formation of hemihydrate. To this end, this study nicely demonstrated that results of high-throughput methods within a DOE study design can be used for systematic investigations of formulation compositions and components that are either beneficial or detrimental for product stability. Data sets, generated by high-throughput approaches, have the benefit of producing greater insights into the most prominent factors that define a design space within which a formulation is providing optimal stability.

Depending on the method design, a typical robustness study can be comprised of between 350 and 1000 samples because the assessment of visual particles requires large sample sets to satisfy statistical constrains on the analysis [2]. Therefore, even though these on Quality by Design (QbD) principle-based multivariate studies increase the sample requirements in comparison to univariate studies, automation of analysis and sample preparation does enable the elucidation of a broader formulation design space, better characterization, and definition of critical quality attributes (CQAs), as well as overall product quality and performance by eliminating very time consuming, human error-prone, hands-on sample handling and operating steps. In support of conducting these types of studies with the representative final drug product configuration, automation options are also available for the handling of the appropriate drug product containers (i.e., vials and syringes). Formulation development activities that support clinical processes like the reconstitution of a lyophilized product for preparation and delivery can benefit from automating the compounding of patient doses for intravenous administration by automation robots [24]. It was shown that robotic compounding could be performed with mAbs without changing the aggregation state of the proteins. Infliximab (Remicade, Janssen Biotech) and trastuzumab (Herceptin, Roche) were studied in lyophilized form, and bevacizumab (Avastin, Roche) as a liquid formulation stored at 2–8°C. The effects of manual and automated reconstitution by a robotic arm (i.v.STATION, Health Robotics) for patient dose preparation on antibody aggregation were evaluated and the influence of vigorous shaking during reconstitution was studied by investigating the propensity of aggregation after rapid aspiration. UV and fluorescence spectroscopy, light scattering, Nile Red fluorescence microscopy, and field-flow fractionation were used to assess aggregation and particulation. The outcome of that study was that samples reconstituted by robotic manipulation had the same aggregation profiles compared with those reconstituted manually. Vials that were vigorously shaken however, showed a significant increase in aggregates. Similarly, rapid aspiration/dispense cycles resulted in a strong increase in aggregation as well. In conclusion, the study demonstrated that robotic systems are gentle enough to achieve reproducible high-quality compounding of various formulations without compromising product quality. These efforts of automation of robotic systems are further supported by a growing trend in the biopharmaceutical industry to develop automation-friendly sample holders and handlers for plate-based high-throughput methods for formulation development and characterization [25]. As an alternative option to plate-based handlers, in an effort to better mimic commercial drug product vial configurations, mini-vial setups can be used for formulation development and optimization, particularly at the later stages of development. These mini vials comply with the dimensional microplate footprint standards that were defined by the Society for Biomolecular Screening

(SBS) in 1995 and can be used with the standard plate holders and autosamplers. The advantage of such a system is that its surface composition closely resembles that of the commercial drug product containers and therefore produces results that are comparable with the results of a traditional single vial platform approach.

Another area that highly benefits from faster chromatography, potentially more than any other area, is analytical method development. In fact, method development is one of the most time-consuming tasks in formulation development. Any acceleration of developing stability-indicating methods for monitoring physical and chemical degradation pathways is significantly accelerating development timelines. With shortening run and analysis times to only a few minutes, adjustments to a method and its parameters can be conducted at a higher cadence. It also provides greater ability to conduct more complex method development by not just rapidly adjusting and refining existing method parameters iteratively, but to screen stationary phases and column resins, different solvents, pH, temperatures, and the slope of the gradient for elution in a much more comprehensive and thorough manner. This in turn enables scientists to develop more reliable and robust methods, which produce data of high quality that qualify for good laboratory practice (GLP) and good manufacturing practice (GMP) requirements. This is an important reality because method transfer into the regulated environment of a Quality laboratory will remain a challenge if the development of high-throughput methods is carried out without GLP and GMP requirements in mind. The key is to develop these high-throughput methods early in development to allow time for method qualification before method transfer to Quality where the methods are validated for release and stability testing. For that, the developed methods have to balance both the need for high-throughput and high-quality analytical standards required by the regulations of GLP and GMP.

The application of automation and high-throughput technologies is starting to be more widely implemented in the biopharmaceutical industry because it is aiding the evaluation of stabilizing solution conditions by permitting a more rapid evaluation of a large matrix of possible combinations, which permits conformational stability and aggregation data to be obtained in a single experiment [26,27]. The quality of these data sets generated by high-throughput methodologies is generally of very high quality because measures of quality control can be easily integrated into high-throughput processes. The use of automated liquid-handling systems significantly decreases the risk of human error during sample preparation. Many quality assurance methods can be used along with automation technologies. Plate pattern recognition [28] and Z′ trend monitoring [29] are methods that help to detect outliers and systematic errors. In addition, improvements in liquid-handling accuracy for low-volume pipetting and dispensing, as well as increased sensitivity of detection, dramatically improve data quality. The notion that the application of high-throughput technologies is expensive and consumes a lot of time may have some merit as the initial stages of high-throughput system setup and testing can be costly and usually takes some time before a system is fully functional and verified. Also the training period of personnel can be quite involved and time consuming. In addition, programming skills are becoming the norm to effectively operate automated instrumentation and robotic workflows in a flexible and reliable way. However, after these initial steps of system setup and training, these high-throughput systems can be run pretty much continuously with a minimum of supervision. High-throughput methodologies are sometimes considered as not very rational or targeted in their application and more often than not are used to apply a so-called "shot gun" approach to formulation development. In reality, given that the experimental approach is sound, high-throughput methodologies allow formulation scientists to generate quality data sets that provide much more complete insights into how formulation components and conditions impact product stability than more traditional experimental designs that are limited by manual sample preparation and low-throughput analytics to fewer components and factors. To obtain such information-rich data sets, broad knowledge of many disciplines is required, including biology, mechanical engineering, computer engineering, and others. For the data to be useful and statistically relevant the development studies need to comply with DOE principles and appropriate sample sizes that allow thorough statistical analysis [30]. More information about data analysis is provided in the next chapter of this book. Taken all the advantages and disadvantages of automation technologies into account, the bottom line is that the reduction in human and systematic error, the increase in efficacies through automation and the generation of more information-rich data sets is worthwhile the initial investment in technology and training. In the end, the upfront investment will be returned by benefiting from shortened development cycle times, improved study execution, and data quality through higher repetition and build-in redundancies, which are normally avoided because of time and resource constrains that come with manual and low-throughput approaches.

Developing a robust and well-defined formulation design space that is ensuring manufacturability, drug performance, and patient safety is associated with significant challenges in terms of resource, materials, experimental complexity of studies and data, as well as ever more aggressive timelines. Traditionally, empirical approaches have been deployed during late-stage and commercial formulation development. They often rely on a trial and error process that is overall inefficient and suboptimal in utilizing material, resources, and time. High-throughput methodologies not only reduce time and resources for formulation development but also create data sets that expedite a more comprehensive understanding about the critical formulation factors that ensure optimal product stability. Striking the right balance between traditional "Quality friendly" non-high-throughput versus high-throughput technologies developed in a timely manner in compliance with Quality requirements and appropriate automation of sample preparation and analysis, can increase the overall throughput, efficiency, consistency, and quality of the development, data, and product.

References

[1] ICH, Pharmaceutical Development Q8(R2), ICH, Geneva, 2004.

[2] K.M. Bower, A. Germansderfer, A. Bruce, B.A. Kerwin, G.R. Kleemann, J.R. Litowski, Designed experiments with binary responses, J. Pharm. Sci. 100 (11) (2011) 5078–5079.

[3] N.W. Warne, Development of high concentration protein biopharmaceuticals: the use of platform approaches in formulation development, Eur. J. Pharm. Biopharm. 78 (2) (2011) 208–212.

[4] D. Low, R. O'Leary, N.S. Pujar, Future of antibody purification, J. Chrom. B 848 (1) (2007) 48–63.
[5] A.A. Shukla, B. Hubbard, T. Tressel, S. Guhan, D. Low, Downstream processing of monoclonal antibodies—application of platform approaches, J. Chrom. B 848 (1) (2007) 28–39.
[6] A. de Villiers, F. Lestremau, R. Szucs, S. Gélébart, F. David, P. Sandra, Evaluation of ultra performance liquid chromatography: Part I. Possibilities and limitations, J. Chrom. A 1127 (1–2) (2006) 60–69.
[7] E. Uliyanchenko, Size-exclusion chromatography-from high-performance to ultra-performance, Anal. Bioanal. Chem. 406 (25) (2014) 6087–6094.
[8] S. Fekete, D. Guillarme, Ultra-high-performance liquid chromatography for the characterization of therapeutic proteins, TrAC Trends Anal. Chem. 63 (2014) 76–84.
[9] D. Chelius, P.V. Bondarenko, Quantitative profiling of proteins in complex mixtures using liquid chromatography and mass spectrometry, J. Proteome Res. 1 (4) (2002) 317–323.
[10] J. Martosella, P. Duong, A. Zhu, Optimising protein and peptide speed and resolution with superficially porous columns, Chrom. Today 6 (2) (2013) 38–40.
[11] S. Molloy, R.M. Fesinmeyer, T. Martinez, D. Murphy Piedmonte, M.E. Pelletier, M.J. Treuheit, et al., Optimized UV detection of high-concentration antibody formulations using high-throughput SE-HPLC, J. Pharm. Sci. (2014). http://dx.doi.org/10.1002/jps.24240.
[12] F. Cilurzo, F. Selmin, P. Minghetti, M. Adami, E. Bertoni, S. Lauria, et al., Injectability evaluation: an open issue, AAPS PharmSciTech 12 (2) (2011) 604–609.
[13] D. Weinbuch, S. Zölls, M. Wiggenhorn, W. Friess, G. Winter, W. Jiskoot, et al., Micro–flow imaging and resonant mass measurement (Archimedes)–complementary methods to quantitatively differentiate protein particles and silicone oil droplets, J. Pharm. Sci. 102 (7) (2013) 2152–2165.
[14] K. Nagamatsu, A. Tomita, Research on the automatic inspection machine of ampoules, J. Takeda Res. Lab. 33 (1974) 43–54.
[15] J. Ge, Y. Wang, B. Zhou, H. Zhang, Intelligent foreign particle inspection machine for injection liquid examination based on modified pulse-coupled neural networks, Sensors 9 (5) (2009) 3386–3404.
[16] F. Strubbe, S. Vandewiele, C. Schreuer, F. Beunis, O. Drobchak, T. Brans, et al., Characterizing and tracking individual colloidal particles using Fourier-Bessel image decomposition, Opt. Express 22 (20) (2014) 24635–24645.
[17] I. Shimizu, F. Kato, A technique for making holograms easily and for measuring simultaneously the behavior of particles of different sizes and/or shapes, Meas. Sci. Technol. 15 (2004) 656–663.
[18] F. Kato, T. Miyakawa, I. Shimizu, Developmental research of visualization of spatial distribution and the behavior of particles in the room, in: Proceedings of 20th Annual Technology Meeting on Air Cleaning and Contamination Control, Tokyo, Japan, 2002.
[19] H. Trnka, J.X. Wu, M.V. De Weert, H. Grohganz, J. Rantanen, Fuzzy logic-based expert system for evaluating cake quality of freeze-dried formulations, J. Pharm. Sci. 102 (12) (2013) 4364–4374.
[20] S. Chandran, V. Nashine, M. Morcos, A. Saluja, A small-scale, material-saving approach to rank-order lyophilized formulations based on reconstitution time, J. Pharm. Innov. 8 (3) (2013) 187–194.
[21] S.K. MacLeod, Moisture determination using Karl Fischer titrations, Anal. Chem. 63 (10) (1991) 557A–566A.

[22] H. Trnka, A. Palou, P.E. Panouillot, A. Kauppinen, M. Toiviainen, H. Grohganz, et al., Near-infrared imaging for high-throughput screening of moisture-induced changes in freeze-dried formulations, J. Pharm. Sci. 103 (9) (2014) 2839–2846.
[23] H.M.L. Larsen, H. Trnka, H. Grohganz, Formation of mannitol hemihydrate in freeze-dried protein formulations—a design of experiment approach, Int. J. Pharm. 460 (1) (2014) 45–52.
[24] B.J. Peters, M.A. Capelle, T. Arvinte, E.M. van de Garde, Validation of an automated method for compounding monoclonal antibody patient doses: case studies of Avastin® (bevacizumab), Remicade® (infliximab) and Herceptin® (trastuzumab), MAbs 5 (1) (2013) 162.
[25] R.E. Majors, New developments in microplates for biological assays and automated sample preparation, LC GC North Am. 22 (11) (2004) 1062–1072.
[26] R. Chaudhuri, Y. Cheng, C.R. Middaugh, D.B. Volkin, High-throughput biophysical analysis of protein therapeutics to examine interrelationships between aggregate formation and conformational stability, AAPS J. 16 (1) (2014) 48–64.
[27] F. He, V.I. Razinkov, C.R. Middaugh, G.W. Becker, High-throughput biophysical approaches to therapeutic protein development, in: L.O. Narhi(Ed.), Biophysics for Therapeutic Protein Development, Biophysics for the Life Sciences, vol. 4, Springer Science+ Business Media, New York, NY, 2013, pp. 7–31. http://dx.doi.org/10.1007/978-1-4614-4316-2_2.
[28] V. Makarenkov, P. Zentilli, D. Kevorkov, A. Gagarin, N. Malo, R. Nadon, An efficient method for the detection and elimination of systematic error in high-throughput screening, Bioinformatics 23 (13) (2007) 1648–1657.
[29] J.H. Zhang, T.D. Chung, K.R. Oldenburg, A simple statistical parameter for use in evaluation and validation of high throughput screening assays, J. Biomol. Screen. 4 (2) (1999) 67–73.
[30] A.O. Grillo, K. Kane, N. Penn, M. Perkins, Characterizing the formulation design space, BioPharm. Int. 23 (3) (2010) 30.

Analysis of high-throughput data

5

5.1 Seeing is believing: the power of data visualization

Even though the examples about the application of automation and high-throughput technologies for formulation design space development provided in the previous chapters are facilitating insights into simple correlations of formulation factors and conditions, the challenge of constructing meaningful correlation models from these complex multidimensional multivariate data sets, however remains. And although multivariate analysis is a mature topic in the field of statistics and despite ample computational power of modern computers, statistical software programs like JMP, SAS, and R have their limits in providing data outputs and visualization tools that allow scientists to easily discern relationships and interactions of factors from more complex data sets. The visualization of data, if used appropriately, allows the organization and presentation of information more intuitively than traditional value tables and two- or three-dimensional graphs and contour plots. It can be a daunting task to make sense of complex data sets if the applied analytical approaches and programs are not capable of discerning the data in a meaningful and obvious way. In fact, the data become meaningless without appropriate organization and presentation.

When using high-throughput screening processes, it is important to keep the various operating steps of a process functional and highly efficient in that the data flow between the individual steps is continuous, seamless, and error-free. Each operating step requires appropriate data processing and visualization for a proper assessment of data quality and further statistical analysis. In addition to controlling data quality, the use of data processing methodologies that are suitable for the analysis, interpretation, and annotation of large data sets is a prerequisite of high-throughput operations. In this section we are reviewing a number of methodologies and tools that are suitable for the analysis of large data sets generated by high-throughput formulation screening campaigns. Additional examples of statistical methods and data processing techniques that allow scientists to better present, visualize, analyze, and interpret complex analytical data sets are discussed in Section 5.2.

The first step to data visualization is the transformation of experimentally obtained raw data into an appropriate data format that is compatible with further analysis. For example, one common type of analysis in formulation studies is size-exclusion high-performance liquid chromatography (SE-HPLC). The data values of a SE-HPLC analysis are obtained by integrating the area of the generated chromatographic peaks. The peak areas can be expressed in absorbance units at a particular wavelength and then be converted into concentrations by knowing the optical path length of the flow cell. This type of data conversion may be useful in cases when a comparison between the protein amount before and after a certain process is required. More commonly however, the

High-Throughput Formulation Development of Biopharmaceuticals. DOI: http://dx.doi.org/10.1016/B978-1-907568-63-3.00005-0

data values generated by a SE-HPLC measurement are presented as relative percentages of integrated peak areas relatively to the integrated total area of all chromatographic peaks. The results are frequently expressed in form of percent change relatively to a reference sample such as the starting material of a stability study. The presentation of relative change is visually distinctive in the cases of ion-exchange high-performance liquid chromatography (IEX-HPLC), where the chromatographic profile is more diverse and comprised of a larger number of peaks. Although spectroscopic data are usually more complex and data rich than chromatographic data, it is not uncommon that raw absorbance and fluorescence spectra reveal little or any differences to the scientist's eye. In such cases, to compare, distinguish, and discover differences between data sets, additional data processing is usually required and greater emphasis needs to be put on data presentation and visualization to aid the process of comprehensive data analysis and interpretation. Advances in computation and graphical representation of data have provided many tools to visualize data in new ways and to allow greater insights and understanding of the results generated within or across different data sets. Constant improvements in computer user interfaces have enhanced the interaction and capabilities for exploring and investigating information visually.

Two-dimensional graphs and tables often become too crowded to show every data point and illustrate trends, correlations, and other behaviors obvious to the human eye. At the same time, elimination or simplification of a data set limits the insight into and comprehension of the data; in a worst-case scenario it may even lead to false or flawed conclusions. If the results are obtained from experiments using a multi-well plate setup (e.g., 96-well plate), a simple table representation can be used, in which every plate well is associated with a value of percentage of monomeric monoclonal antibody (mAb) that was determined by SE-HPLC for each formulation after incubation at elevated temperature (Fig. 5.1A). Furthermore, to make the presentation and meaning of the values more perceptive, every value can be associated with a color code to enhance the visualization of the results and make the presentation of the data more intuitive for the human eye. For example, in Fig. 5.1B, higher levels of aggregation, which correlates with a loss in main peak area, expressed here in percent main peak, are indicated by the color red. Lower aggregation values that correlate with no or only a small loss in main peak area are presented with the color green. These so-called "heat maps" help the formulation scientists to quickly and intuitively identify well-performing formulations from those that do not stabilize the protein product. Another way to present the same data set is to use a three-dimensional bar graph in which the height of the bars corresponds proportionally to the amount of monomeric molecule (Fig. 5.1C). In Fig. 5.1B, comparing the aggregation levels across the table columns reveals that the level of aggregation is the lowest in every third column, implying that the formulation composition for these columns is providing the greatest stability. The visual examination of complex data sets is useful and necessary to exclude obvious artifacts as early as possible. The advantage of applying appropriate visualization programs and presentations to large data sets, generated by high-throughput processes, lies in the opportunity and ability to look at an entire data set as a whole, comprehensively at once. This approach avoids oversimplification of the data analysis and presentation by using tabulations or graphical representations with limited resolution and dimensions.

(A)

	1	2	3	4	5	6	7	8	9	10	11	12
A	27.9	15.0	24.4	11.8	10.8	30.5	91.8	91.6	91.8	91.6	91.3	91.5
B	95.0	95.3	95.4	95.0	95.1	95.7	95.2	95.1	95.8	95.4	94.2	95.6
C	93.6	93.5	95.3	93.6	93.4	95.6	92.6	92.4	95.5	93.0	91.0	94.6
D	8.1	7.2	74.6	11.1	8.0	79.1	85.3	85.2	90.5	86.7	85.0	90.8
E	94.7	93.6	95.0	94.8	94.3	95.2	95.1	95.2	95.0	95.4	94.7	95.4
F	94.0	94.0	95.7	92.8	93.7	95.8	94.6	95.3	95.4	94.7	94.4	95.9
G	93.9	93.5	94.3	93.7	92.3	95.2	93.9	93.2	94.7	94.2	93.2	94.9
H	87.3	86.7	94.3	90.5	89.6	94.3	90.4	90.9	93.7	92.2	91.7	93.8

(B)

	1	2	3	4	5	6	7	8	9	10	11	12
A	27.9	15.0	24.4	11.8	10.8	30.5	91.8	91.6	91.8	91.6	91.3	91.5
B	95.0	95.3	95.4	95.0	95.1	95.7	95.2	95.1	95.8	95.4	94.2	95.6
C	93.6	93.5	95.3	93.6	93.4	95.6	92.6	92.4	95.5	93.0	91.0	94.6
D	8.1	7.2	74.6	11.1	8.0	79.1	85.3	85.2	90.5	86.7	85.0	90.8
E	94.7	93.6	95.0	94.8	94.3	95.2	95.1	95.2	95.0	95.4	94.7	95.4
F	94.0	94.0	95.7	92.8	93.7	95.8	94.6	95.3	95.4	94.7	94.4	95.9
G	93.9	93.5	94.3	93.7	92.3	95.2	93.9	93.2	94.7	94.2	93.2	94.9
H	87.3	86.7	94.3	90.5	89.6	94.3	90.4	90.9	93.7	92.2	91.7	93.8

(C)

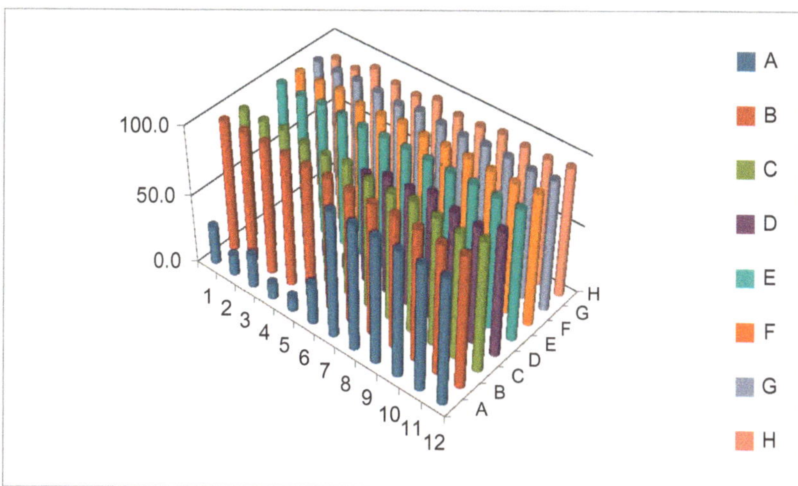

Figure 5.1 Graphical representation of high-throughput data obtained by SE-HPLC of a monoclonal antibody molecule in 96 different formulations after incubation at elevated temperature. The percentage of SE-HPLC main peak area is shown as a plain table (A), color-coded "heat map" table (B), and three-dimensional bar graph (C).

An interesting and effective way to work with multivariate data sets has been proposed by researchers from the University of Kansas [1]. Kalonia's researchers are using radar chart array analysis to visualize data sets generated by multiple analytical techniques to identify the effects of formulation variables on the formulation of particles of an IgG1 mAb drug product formulation. In their study the data of aggregation and particulation measurements, performed by SE-HPLC, micro-flow imaging (MFI), and Archimedes resonant mass measurements, were arranged and plotted as radar charts. A radar chart, also known as a spider chart or a star chart, because of its appearance, is able to display multivariate data in the form of a two-dimensional chart of three or more quantitative variables represented on separate axes starting from the same point in the center of the chart. In this particular case, radar charts were created to visualize mAb aggregation and particle formation by combining data sets from different analytical methods (Fig. 5.2). Different conditions, like pH and salt concentrations, were found to affect the size and morphology of aggregates, which were easily recognizable by the way they were illustrated by the radar charts.

As heat resistance is a proxy for long-term aggregation propensity of proteins, thermal stability assays are routinely performed using various spectroscopic and light

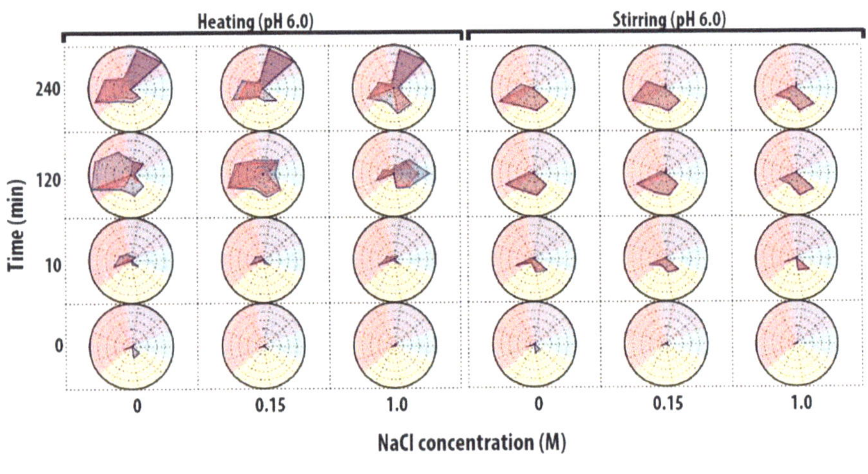

Figure 5.2 Radar chart array analysis of subvisible particle concentration and size data for IgG1 mAb solutions as measured by MFI. IgG1 mAb solutions of varying pH values and NaCl concentrations were exposed to different stress types over time as indicated in the figure (n = 3). The resulting formation of subvisible particles was measured by MFI. The *Y*-axis represents the amount of time the formulations were stressed (in minutes), the *X*-axis represents NaCl concentrations, and each radar chart panel (left, middle, and right) signifies a change in stress or pH. The different angles on the charts represent different sizes of subvisible particles.
Source: From C. Kalonia, O.S. Kumru, J.H. Kim, C.R. Middaugh, D.B. Volkin, Radar chart array analysis to visualize effects of formulation variables on IgG1 particle formation as measured by multiple analytical techniques, J. Pharm. Sci. 102 (12) (2013) 4256–4267, Figure 2.

scattering detection methods. To increase the throughput of thermal stability analysis, Boulet-Audet et al. [2] introduced macro attenuated total reflection Fourier transform infrared (ATR-FTIR) spectroscopic imaging as a novel method for high-throughput thermal stability analysis of mAbs. This chemically specific visualization method has the distinct advantage of being able to discriminate between monomeric and aggregated proteins. The method creates an image that is generated by the IR amide II band area of the Fourier transform infrared (FTIR) spectra of protein samples with different buffer compositions on a 12-well plate. The ATR-FTIR images of the high-throughput grid were measured using a cooled mercury cadmium telluride (MCT) focal plane array displaying 128 by 128 elements, resulting in 16,384 simultaneous infrared spectra. The images were aggregated to 64 by 64 by averaging groups of 4 pixels to reduce memory requirements. The infrared spectra with pixel positions corresponding to the bottom of each of the 12 wells were averaged and reduced to a single variable proportional to the local protein concentration at the bottom layer of the wells by integrating the amide II band between 1590 and 1495 cm^{-1}. To visualize the IgG aggregation kinetic, the difference in absorbance of the amide II band was plotted as a function of time.

But even these types of more sophisticated visualization techniques fall short in their ability to visualize and quantify existing correlations for even more complex data sets. To determine whether a difference between control sample and a number of test samples that have been exposed to a variety of different conditions is significant or just caused by pure chance, it is necessary to perform thorough statistical analyses with the aid of more state-of-the-art visualization techniques. Analytics platforms like TIBCO Spotfire, Tableau, Qlik, and others provide comprehensive and feature-rich analytics and visualization tools that leverage S+ or R programming language engines to solve problems in modeling and predictions, pattern detection, and optimization. Visualization of complex data sets facilitates greater clarity that allows the discovery of patterns, trends, gaps, and outliers; in other words a more comprehensive insight into the underlying meaning, correlations, and significance of complex multivariate data sets. To this end, the next section is devoted to the application of additional statistical and visualization tools.

5.2 Making sense of high-throughput screening and multidimensional characterization

This section describes the application of statistical tools and challenges in statistical data analysis related to high-throughput screening processes that are comprised of appropriately powered experimental designs, statistical analyses, and the interpretation of data to aid the decision making process of selecting a formulation or formulation space that is most suitable for a protein drug product. In the field of protein formulation development, the analysis of multivariable behavior and the construction of models for quantifying correlations among a large number of variables are fundamentally important for accurately predicting shelf-life stability. The stability of a protein during storage depends on the inherent properties of the protein, the conditions it is exposed to (e.g., temperature, pH, ionic strength, agitation), and cosolute concentrations of the solvent. It is desirable to identify the critical factors that significantly affect protein solubility and stability from empirically collected data and identify correlations and interactions that contribute to the observed behaviors. Therefore, the major part of experimental planning is to decide which input conditions need to be introduced and which output responses are to be recorded. Since the formulation design space and the monitored behavioral characteristics of a given biotherapeutic are a consequence of these many factors, multivariate analysis is necessary and multivariate data must be examined in the context of all factors simultaneously. Therefore, the inherent complexity of multivariate studies and analyses is making high-throughput experimental design the methodology of choice. As mentioned in Chapter 1, High-throughput methodology in biopharmaceutical formulation development, the first step of high-throughput data analysis involves the experimental design of a variety of studies and experiments. The principles of design of experiments (DOE) have been successfully applied by many industries including the biopharmaceutical industry. The US Food and Drug Administration (FDA) instituted several initiatives to facilitate the implementation of robust manufacturing processes and the production of high quality biopharmaceuticals [3]. The concept of Quality by Design (QbD) includes DOE principles [4] as an essential part of scientific planning and execution. Due to the multitude of factors that describe a formulation design space, formulation components should be screened simultaneously to enable the accurate identification of the critical factors and their interactions that provide optimal stability. For the design of formulation screening studies, the factors that need to be evaluated are dependent on the molecule, the phase of development, and the maturity of the manufacturing process. For the most part, protein properties, as well as process and manufacture requirements dictate the extent and complexity of formulation development studies. For certain well-characterized and inherently stable molecules, with a rich historical experience, formulation platforms can be deployed to minimize development work and limit drug product formulation development to a verification exercise. In the early phases of development, the experimental design may need to be adjusted to the limited availability of material and a larger pool of molecule candidates. In addition, the manufacturing experience is still variable and often quite limited during this stage, as, for example, purification operations such as ultrafiltration–diafiltration used to formulate the product may result in pH and excipient levels that differ from the target formulation [5,6]. In such cases, the limited input for initial formulation development studies may force formulation scientists to predict and focus on the most critical factors and appropriate stability indicating analytical methods, while setting the ranges and concentrations of formulation factors relatively wide to be inclusive of the desired formulation design space. In certain instances, when operating with a class of similar molecules, historical data and information can be used to set the initial target ranges and concentrations of formulation factors. For late-stage development, when the final dosage form, the commercial formulation, and device configuration are being finalized, the focus is shifting to demonstrating that the final formulation candidate is stable within the given robustness parameters and to understand a drug product formulation's tolerability toward process variability.

There are many types and subtypes of experimental designs that are applicable for formulation screening studies [7]. Depending on the number of experimental design and response factors the experimental designs vary from screening designs to response surface and full factorial designs. Fractional factorial designs are appropriate when the resources are limited and not all interactions between response factors are significant or fully understood. The stability providing response factors that are significant, as well as the factor levels and ranges can be determined and optimized with the help of surface response designs such as central composite and Box–Behnken designs. In both designs the curvature of the response surface is determined by building a second-order (quadratic) model for the response variables without needing to use a complete three-level factorial experiment, which decreases the number of required experiments. In the case studies presented by Grillo et al. [8], the robustness of lyophilized and liquid formulations were tested using partial factorial designs. The values of protein concentration, buffer concentration, pH, surfactant, and cryo/lyoprotectant were deviated from the target values to monitor the changes in aggregation rates at different temperatures. In case of the lyophilized formulations, robustness was demonstrated by showing that variations of these values within the levels of the formulation design space had only a minimal or no impact on product quality, whereas for the liquid formulation, formulation components were identified that required to be tightly controlled.

In the following paragraph, an example is presented, in which high-throughput screening and analysis methodologies were combined on one hand to comprehensively screen a high number of formulation factors and storage conditions, and on the other hand to determine their significance by applying statistical analysis of the corresponding responses that were measured. Each response could be or could not be dependent on the formulation factors part of the screening matrix. Therefore, it is imperative to distinguish the significant correlations from random, insignificant response values that do not represent a relevant signal. The more data points are analyzed the better is the signal-to-noise ratio and the accuracy of predicting a response value. In one example, 81 different mAb formulations were screened to determine two important characterization factors: (1) thermal stability and (2) viscosity [9]. As previously mentioned in Chapter 2, both high viscosity and low thermal stability can be limiting factors for drug development. The correct selection of formulation components can improve the solution properties of an antibody formulation. However, it is possible that the same formulation factors may induce opposite effects on viscosity and thermal stability. It has been shown that addition of salt in some cases can decrease the viscosity of protein formulations [10] but at the same time it also significantly decreased a protein's thermal stability [11].

To find the optimal formulation conditions, it is necessary to understand the correlation between both the molecular parameters and formulation factors. To this end, He et al. [9] used two high-throughput methods to measure thermal stability and viscosity of a variety of formulations. The measured temperature of hydrophobic exposure T_h, measured by differential scanning fluorescence (DSF), correlated well with the melting temperature T_m, determined by differential scanning calorimetry (DSC) [12]. Therefore, both T_m and T_h served as parameters for thermal stability.

Formulation viscosity was determined by a dynamic light scattering (DLS) method that was described in Chapter 2 [13]. The formulation factors that were assessed included pH 5.0, 5.5, and 6.0, protein concentrations of 90, 120, and 150 mg/mL, the presence of sucrose or proline, and the presence of Ca^{2+} or Mg^{2+} ions. The screening matrix was a 3^4 full factorial design and the data were analyzed using multivariate correlation tools provided by the JMP software (SAS Institute Inc., Cary, North Carolina). The prediction model took only significant factors into account and the significance of those factors was determined along with their level of contribution to the response value. Basically a second-order polynomial equation was constructed using all factors, numerical and categorical, and interactions between them. Then the equation was fitted to experimental data points by a least square method. The resulting best-fit expression was:

$$Y = b_1 x_1 + b_2 x_2 + b_1 x_1 x_2 + \cdots + b_n x_n + b_{nm} x_n x_m + b_k x_n^2 + \varepsilon(error) \quad (5.1)$$

where Y is the response, x is a formulation factor, and b is a coefficient that could be used to estimate the level of each factor's contribution; b can also be called the *parameter estimate*. For categorical factors each separate coefficient corresponds to a separate factor. The coefficient ε is an error indicating the difference between predicted and actual data. As soon as a prediction model is constructed, there is a good opportunity to explore the landscape of responses within the coordinates of the tested formulation factors. In Figs. 5.3 and 5.4, viscosity and T_h values are plotted as contour plots in pH and protein concentration coordinates. Different shades of gray correspond to specific viscosity values (Fig. 5.3) starting from < 4 cP (white area) to > 12 cP (black area). The values beyond that range are not shown. The contour plots are created for various combinations of sucrose and Ca^{2+} concentrations in antibody formulations. The contour surfaces are shown in 1 cP intervals and the gradient of viscosity can be tracked for each condition. In fact, the gradient can be very useful in the evaluation of robustness, when the changes in response are measured against small changes in formulation factors. Similar to terrain maps, the slope of response values in the direction of coordinate changes is representative of stability. As shown in Fig. 5.3, for samples without ions the slope for viscosity is becoming increasingly steeper when the values approach 12 cP. The addition of Ca^{2+} ions, on the other hand, decreases the viscosity and results in a viscosity landscape that is more flat, while the presence of sucrose induces a slight increase in viscosity. Similar to the viscosity prediction model data, thermostability data were also converted to contour plots (Fig. 5.4). In contrast to viscosity, thermostability contours shown in Fig. 5.4 depend mainly on pH and not on protein concentration, although a slight increase in slope is observed at higher pH values. Both sucrose and Ca^{2+} ions significantly change T_h but in opposite directions. Sucrose shifts the T_h values to higher temperatures, whereas Ca^{2+} ions reduce the formulation T_h to lower values. In addition to their utility to map out a drug's formulation design space, contour plots are also useful for the identification and optimization of formulations that provide optimal stability and manufacturability properties. The DOE concept described here [9] serves as a case illustration for how statistical tools can be applied to find a compromise between

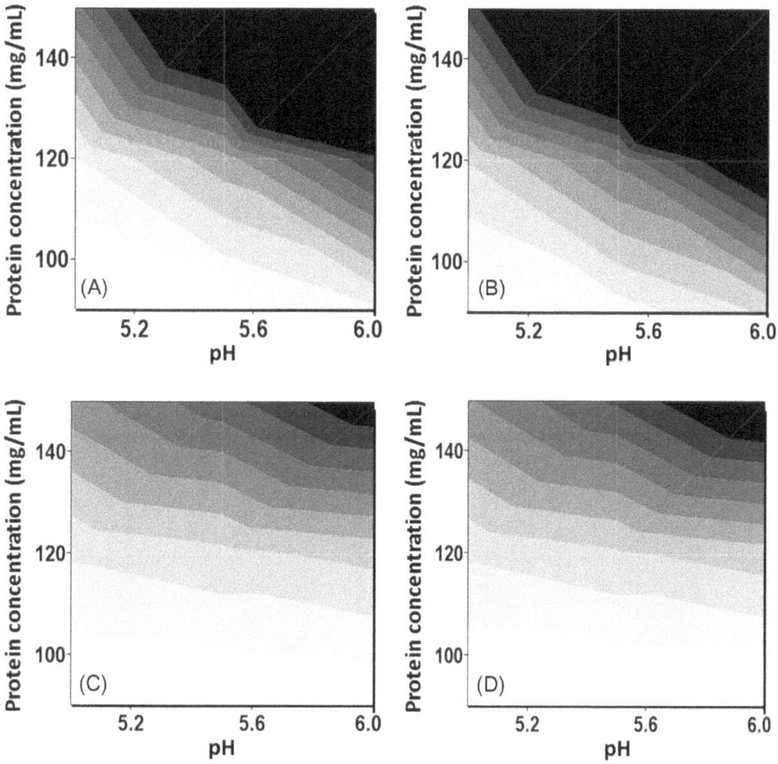

Figure 5.3 Contour plots for the prediction models of viscosity values for various formulation conditions. The same shade of gray corresponds to the same value of viscosity. The white color area indicates viscosity values below 4 cP, while the black color area indicates values higher than 12 cP. The difference between the individual shades is 1 cP. (A) no ions + no excipients, (B) no ions + sucrose, (C) Ca^{2+} ions + no excipients, (D) Ca^{2+} ions + sucrose.

conflicting formulation factors affecting two response parameters. In this particular case the two responses, T_h and viscosity, were optimized to influence the effects on these responses in opposite directions, i.e., increasing T_h and decreasing viscosity. To this end, it is necessary to determine the factors that result in high thermostability and low viscosity. In Fig. 5.5, contour plots are shown for both T_h and viscosity as a function of four different combinations of excipient and ion concentrations. The minimum allowed T_h value was selected to be 50°C (blue line) and the maximum allowed value for viscosity was selected to be 6 cP (red line). The areas with a T_h lower than 50°C and a viscosity higher than 6 cP are shown in blue and red, respectively. The areas of the desired response values are white. According to the contour plots a formulation without excipients and ions is limited by a protein concentration of 120 mg/mL at pH 5.25 (Fig. 5.5A). The presence of the excipient sucrose allows for an expanded pH range down to 5.0, while still achieving a T_h > 50°C, but at the same time requires a

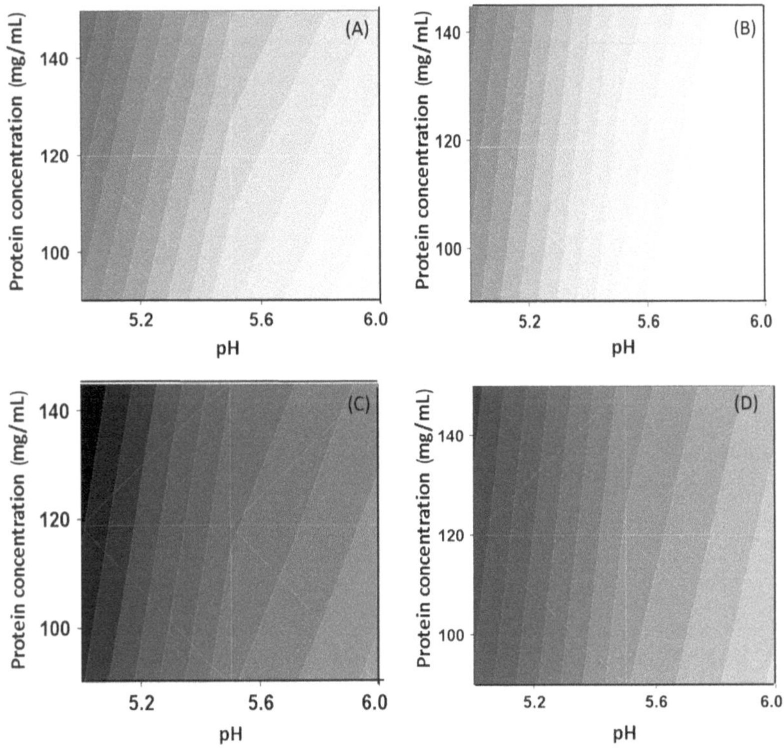

Figure 5.4 Contour plots for the prediction models of T_h values for various formulation conditions. The same shade of gray corresponds to the same value of T_h. The white color area indicates T_h values higher than 55°C, while the black color area indicates values below 45°C. The difference between the individual shades is 1°C. (A) no ions + no excipients, (B) no ions + sucrose, (C) Ca^{2+} ions + no excipients, (D) Ca^{2+} ions + sucrose.

slightly lower protein concentration to achieve a viscosity < 6 cP (Fig. 5.5B). On the other hand, the addition of Ca^{2+} ions in the absence of an excipient leaves no room for an acceptable range of pH values and protein concentrations, mainly because of low T_h values < 50°C (Fig. 5.5C). In Fig. 5.5D, the profiler is shown for the samples with sucrose and with the addition of Ca^{2+} ions. In this case, the allowable range of protein concentrations is still approximately the same as shown in Fig. 5.5B (< 120 mg/mL) but the acceptable range of pH values is narrower and closer to the higher values evaluated in this study (pH > 5.5).

He et al. [14] focused on the thermal and colloidal stability of various IgG antibody formulations to define an optimal formulation design space that minimizes the propensity of aggregate formation. Thermal stability was explored by DSF measurements and colloidal stability was estimated by the interaction parameter k_D measured by a high-throughput DLS method. In addition to the measurements of T_h and k_D, the aggregation propensities were measured under accelerated aggregation conditions to verify the predictive accuracy of these parameters. Aggregation was induced

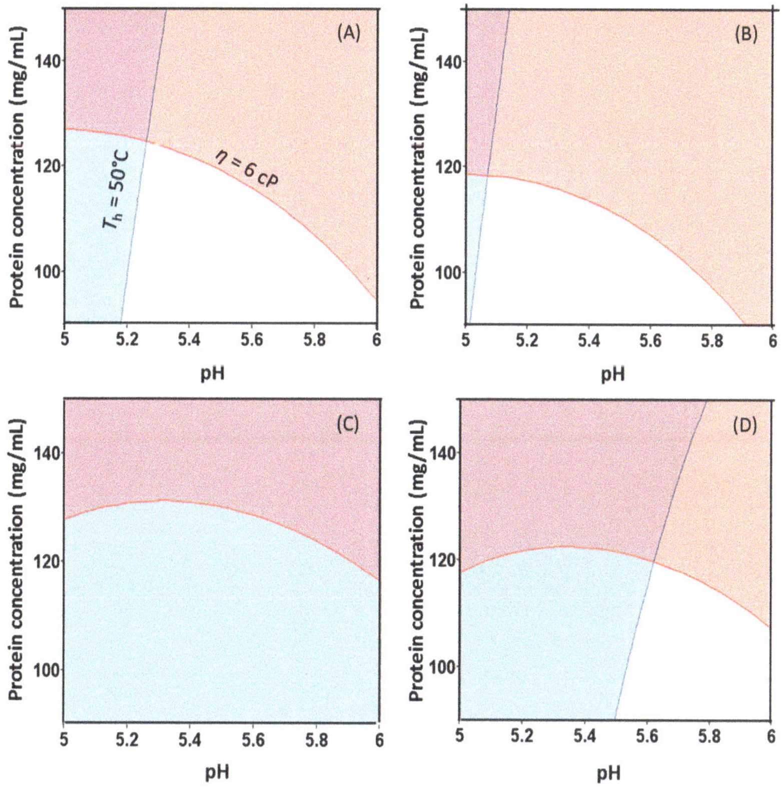

Figure 5.5 Contour profilers derived from prediction formulas for T_h and viscosity values. The areas in white are shown as acceptable at particular limits for T_h and viscosity values. The low T_h value limit is 50°C and the high viscosity value is 6 cP. Areas with acceptable pH and protein concentrations are shown for the following formulations: (A) no ions + no excipients, (B) no ions + sucrose, (C) Ca^{2+} ions + no excipients, (D) Ca^{2+} ions + sucrose. T_h, temperature of hydrophobic exposure.
Source: From F. He, C.E. Woods, E. Trilisky, K.M. Bower, J.R. Litowski, B.A. Kerwin, et al., Screening of monoclonal antibody formulations based on high-throughput thermostability and viscosity measurements: design of experiment and statistical analysis, J. Pharm. Sci. 100 (4) (2011) 1330–1340, Figure 4.

by high temperature and mechanical agitation. After agitation, large particles were the major component of the aggregated fraction and they were counted by relatively low-throughput MFI, limiting the number of formulations to just 21. In this study it was important to understand how the two stability indicating parameters depend on what type of formulation factors and whether or not these factors were benefiting from both, either or, or none of the two stability parameters. The same type of prediction modeling used in the previously described study [9] was applied in this work to determine the effect of formulation factors and conditions on the colloidal and thermal stability parameters. Contour plots helped to illustrate a thermal stability profile

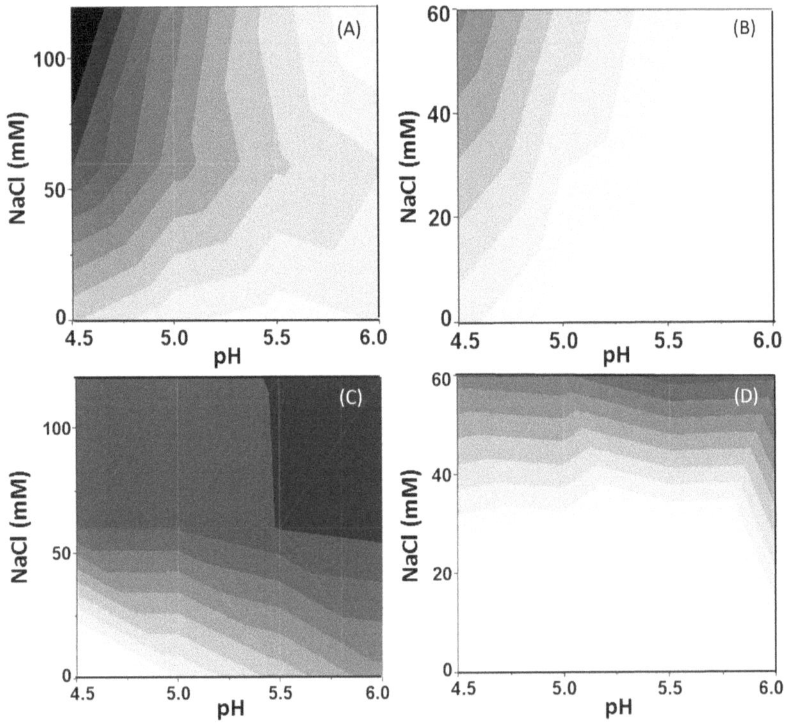

Figure 5.6 Contour plots for the prediction models of T_h values under various formulation conditions (A) without excipients and (B) with sucrose. The same shade of gray corresponds to the same value of T_h and k_D. The white color areas in the T_h contour plots (A and B) indicate T_h values higher than 55°C, while the black color areas indicate the T_h values below 45°C. The difference between the individual shades is 1°C. Contour plots for the predicted models of k_D values under various formulation conditions (C) without excipients and (D) with sucrose. The white color areas in the k_D contour plots (C and D) indicate the k_D values higher than 40 mL/g, while the black color areas indicate the values below −10 mL/g.
Source: From F. He, C.E. Woods, G.W. Becker, L.O. Narhi, V.I. Razinkov, High-throughput assessment of thermal and colloidal stability parameters for monoclonal antibody formulations, J. Pharm. Sci. 100 (12) (2011) 5126–5141, Figure 9.

(Fig. 5.6) that indicated a strong T_h dependency on both NaCl concentration and pH. The addition of sucrose shifted T_h values toward higher temperatures (Fig. 5.6B). Sucrose also changed the k_D profile by making the IgG formulations less dependent on pH and generally more colloidally stable (Fig. 5.6D). Interestingly, in the absence of sucrose, the T_h profile split into two high temperature areas, one at high pH and the other at high NaCl concentrations. The critical values for each parameter were selected based on aggregation data obtained during protein-stress studies. It was found that aggregation levels increased significantly at temperatures higher than 52°C (Fig. 5.7). Protein-agitation studies showed that for k_D values below 7 mL/g the number of particles caused by agitation increased by several orders of magnitude (Fig. 5.8).

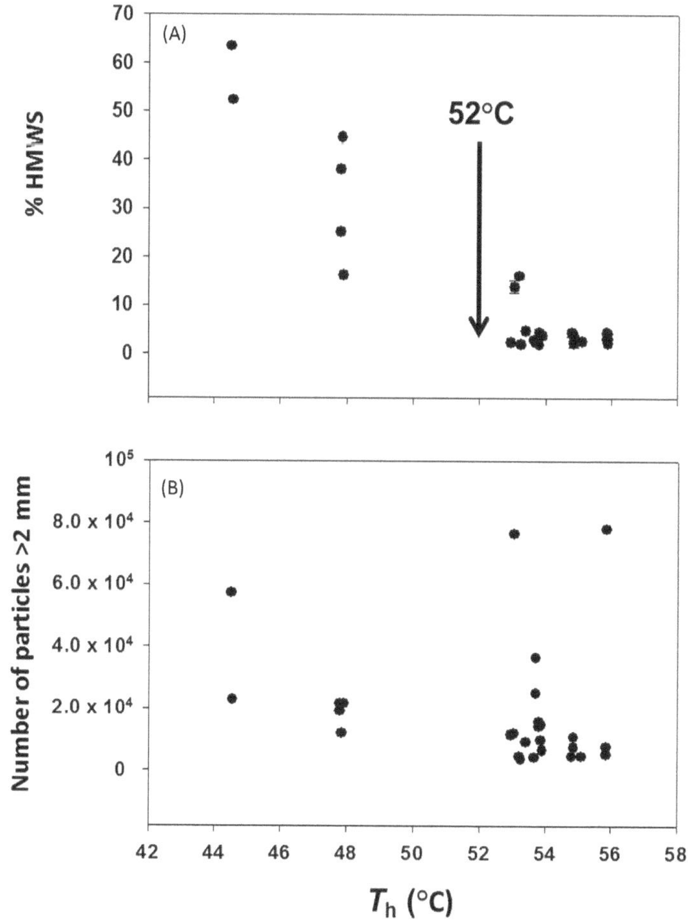

Figure 5.7 (A) The percentage of high molecular weight species (HMWS) obtained after thermal stress is shown as a function of the experimental T_h values. (B) The number of particles per milliliter after thermal stress is shown versus T_h values for each formulation. *Source*: From F. He, C.E. Woods, G.W. Becker, L.O. Narhi, V.I. Razinkov, High-throughput assessment of thermal and colloidal stability parameters for monoclonal antibody formulations, J. Pharm. Sci. 100 (12) (2011) 5126–5141, Figure 4.

In Fig. 5.9, contour profiles are shown that predict T_h and k_D values as a function of pH and salt concentrations. The contour plots nicely illustrate that if T_h is raised from 52°C to 54°C, the stability profile changes dramatically to the point that stable formulation conditions are limited to a small area defined by very low salt concentrations (close to zero) and pH values between 5.0 and 6.0 (Fig. 5.9C). However, the addition of sucrose can restore some of the formulation stability even at 54°C (Fig. 5.9D).

Another example of a high-throughput assessment of protein stability is presented by the work of Alekseychyk et al. [15]. The employment of high-throughput stress

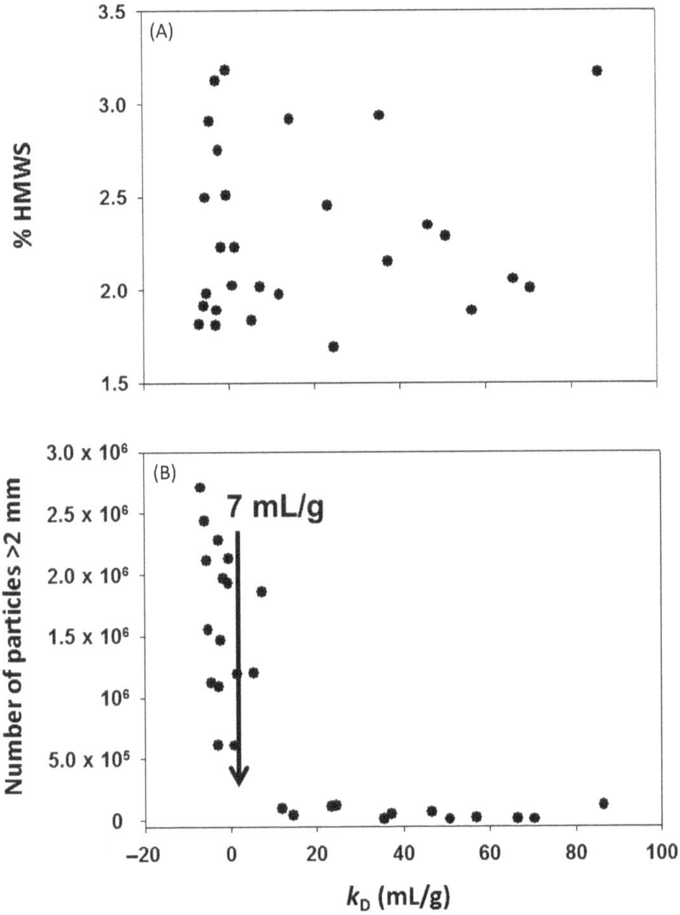

Figure 5.8 (A) The percentage of high molecular weight species (HMWS) after mechanical stress versus k_D values. (B) The number of particles per milliliter after mechanical stress versus k_D values.
Source: From F. He, C.E. Woods, G.W. Becker, L.O. Narhi, V.I. Razinkov, High-throughput assessment of thermal and colloidal stability parameters for monoclonal antibody formulations, J. Pharm. Sci. 100 (12) (2011) 5126–5141, Figure 7.

studies and characterization analytics utilizing a 96-well plate-based study approach, allowed the screening of a large number of formulations and the identification of the most stabilizing formulation conditions. To this end, a full factorial formulation study of 96 formulations of antistreptavidin antibodies (an IgG1 and an IgG2) and various high-throughput stress (elevated temperatures) and characterization techniques were conducted to select the most stable formulations. The analytical methods applied in this study were all 96-well plate-based using an automated liquid-handling system (Tecan) to prepare the different formulations and sample plates. Ninety-six

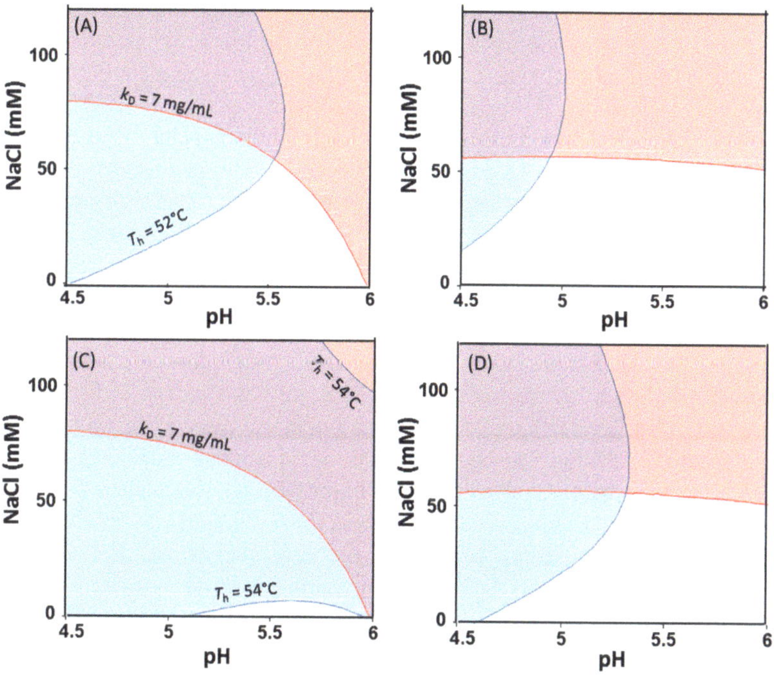

Figure 5.9 Contour profiles derived from prediction formulas for T_h and k_D values. The areas in white represent the acceptable values of pH and salt concentrations at the particular limits for T_h and k_D. The areas with T_h values < 52°C (A and B) and T_h values < 54°C (C and D) are shown in red. The areas with k_D < 7.0 mL/g are shown in blue. The areas with acceptable pH and salt concentrations are shown for the formulations without excipients (A and C) and with sucrose (B and D).

Source: From F. He, C.E. Woods, G.W. Becker, L.O. Narhi, V.I. Razinkov, High-throughput assessment of thermal and colloidal stability parameters for monoclonal antibody formulations, J. Pharm. Sci. 100 (12) (2011) 5126–5141, Figure 10.

formulation samples were prepared by the automatic liquid-handling system in two 48-well plates of 3 mL per well volume. Then the formulations were distributed in smaller volumes (150–200 μL) to 96-well plates, each of which were assigned to specific stress or analytical methods. The advantage of this methodology is that it only requires a small number and variety of plates and plate types, respectively. For example, the plates, which were sealed and incubated at elevated temperature, could be unsealed and transferred directly to the autosampler of the ultra-performance liquid chromatography system for analysis by size-exclusion ultra-performance liquid chromatography (SE-UPLC) without any further sample preparation. The content of each plate could be quickly and easily distributed to other plates with the help of the automated liquid-handling system. Mechanical agitation and high-temperature incubation were used as the stress methods to test both the propensity of aggregation and fragmentation (i.e., protein backbone cleavage). Before each stress study, conformational stability was evaluated by DSF. The temperature of hydrophobic exposure (T_h) was determined for each formulation at the midpoint of the lowest temperature transition from the first derivative of the fluorescence signal over a temperature range from 20°C to 95°C. The values of the integrated peak areas of the SE-UPLC main peak (monomeric antibody), high molecular weight and low molecular weight peaks were determined after application of the thermal and mechanical stress methods. Multivariate regression analysis of high-throughput data was performed to find statistically significant formulation factors that alter measured parameters such as the percentage of monomeric antibody or unfolding temperature. The data were analyzed using multivariate correlation tools provided by JMP software (SAS Institute Inc., Cary, North Carolina). As described earlier [9], the prediction model takes only significant factors into account and the significance of those factors can be determined along with the level of contribution to the response values. Basically the second-order polynomial equation was constructed using all factors, numerical and categorical, and interactions between them (Eq. (5.1)). Two output response parameters were measured in the study. First, the temperature of hydrophobic exposure (T_h) obtained by DSF and second, the percentage of integrated main peak area obtained by high-throughput SE-UPLC after incubation at 40°C and mechanical agitation. For each output response that was derived from different formulation conditions—various formulation factors such as pH, excipients, and the presence of salt or detergent—a multivariate regression model was constructed for T_h and monomeric antibody. The prediction model was constructed using a multivariate correlation method and the predicted values were compared with the measured values by plotting them on a "Predicted versus Actual" graph. In Fig. 5.10A and B the experimentally determined T_h values are plotted against the predicted T_h for the investigated IgG1 and IgG2 antistreptavidin antibodies. The linearity of the plots, described by the R^2 parameter as a root-mean-square error or the generalized distance of the data points from the linear regression line, indicates the goodness of our constructed models. The found correlation polynomial equation can serve as an analytical expression to find response values under specific conditions in specific formulations, and therefore enables the selection of the formulations with maximal thermal stability based on predicted T_h values. In Fig. 5.11, the T_h dependence on pH is shown for various formulations. As it is indicated in the figure, maximum thermal stability was predicted for a pH range between pH 5.5 and pH 6.0 for acetate buffer and between pH 6.7 and pH 7.1 for phosphate buffer. The presence of salt had the most significant effect on T_h. The difference between T_h values for IgG1 and IgG2 antibodies was the greatest at low pH and becoming virtually nonexistent at pH > 6.0. In conclusion, the presented prediction model is providing a complete picture of thermal stability of both IgG1 and IgG2 antibodies in all of the 96 formulations investigated. In addition, conformational stability was correlated to the levels of degradation caused by heating or agitation. To this end, the 96-well plates with antibody formulations were either incubated for 2 weeks at 4°C, 25°C, and 40°C, or exposed to mechanical agitation stress for 24 hours at 4°C using an orbital shaker. The level of degradation was measured by SE-UPLC with the percentage of integrated main peak area (monomeric antibody) serving as the output value in the regression models. No significant changes in the percentages of

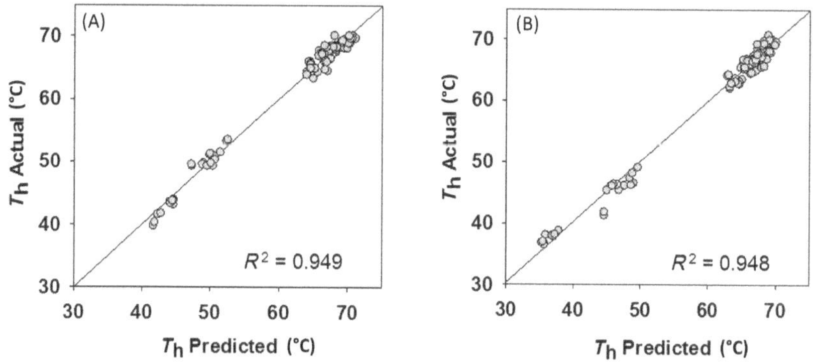

Figure 5.10 Experimentally determined T_h values plotted against predicted T_h values for IgG1 (A) and IgG2 (B) antistreptavidin molecules.
Source: From L. Alekseychyk, C. Su, G.W. Becker, M.J. Treuheit, V.I. Razinkov, High-throughput screening and stability optimization of anti-streptavidin IgG1 and IgG2 formulations, J. Biomol. Screen. 19 (9) (2014) 1290–1301, Figure 1.

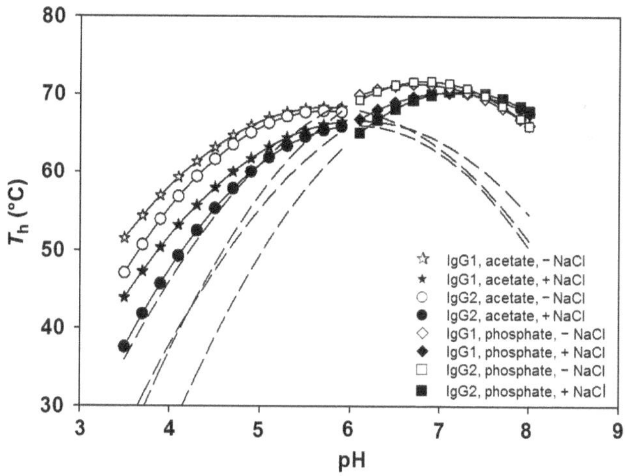

Figure 5.11 T_h dependence on pH for antistreptavidin antibodies predicted by multivariate analysis of differential scanning fluorimetry (DSF) data. The results are shown for IgG1 (stars, diamonds), IgG2 (circles, squares), acetate buffer (stars, circles), and phosphate buffer (diamonds, squares); formulations without salt, open symbols; formulations with salt, filled symbols. Dashed lines correspond to extrapolated data. All data are shown for formulations without detergent and with proline as an excipient.
Source: From L. Alekseychyk, C. Su, G.W. Becker, M.J. Treuheit, V.I. Razinkov, High-throughput screening and stability optimization of anti-streptavidin IgG1 and IgG2 formulations, J. Biomol. Screen. 19 (9) (2014) 1290–1301, Figure 1.

monomeric antibody were found after mechanical agitation at 4°C and incubation at 4°C and 25°C. Only incubation at 40°C resulted in significant degradation of monomeric antibodies and significant correlations between percent peak area and the assessed formulation factors. The same modeling technique was applied to correlate changes in pH to conformational stability or the level of degradation measured by SE-UPLC (Fig. 5.12A and B). Interestingly, the shapes of the percent monomer plots are similar to the plots describing the T_h model. The maxima of percent monomer are

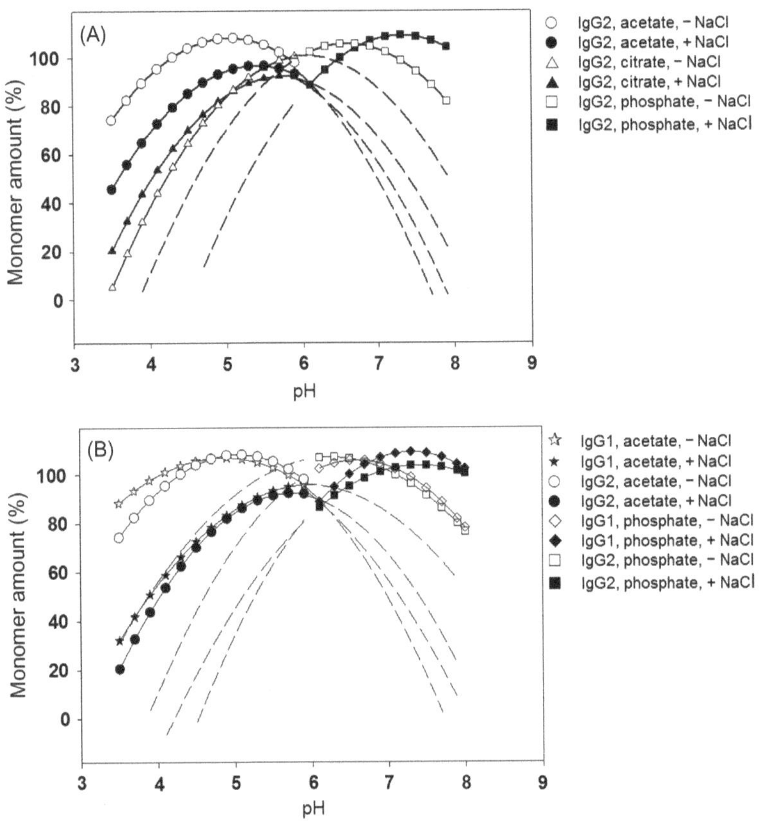

Figure 5.12 (A) Predicted functions for antistreptavidin IgG2 monomer amount obtained by SE-UPLC and plotted as a function of pH. The functions are presented for acetate (circles), citrate (triangles), and phosphate (squares) buffers in the presence (filled symbols) and absence (open symbols) of salt. The dashed lines indicate a pH range beyond the experimental conditions for a particular function. (B) Predicted functions for antistreptavidin monomer amount plotted as a function of pH. The functions are presented for acetate (stars, circles) and phosphate (diamonds, squares) buffers in the presence (filled symbols) and absence (open symbols) of salt for IgG1 (stars and diamonds) and IgG2 (circles and squares). *Source*: From L. Alekseychyk, C. Su, G.W. Becker, M.J. Treuheit, V.I. Razinkov, High-throughput screening and stability optimization of anti-streptavidin IgG1 and IgG2 formulations, J. Biomol. Screen. 19 (9) (2014) 1290–1301, Figure 2.

located in approximately the same pH range as the maxima for the T_h functions, which were derived from the DSF data. The data that were predicted beyond the tested formulation parameters are indicated by the dashed lines. Besides the similar responses of percent monomer and T_h to changes in pH, the plots also indicate that the presence of salt shifts the maxima toward higher pH values. The maxima of percent monomer are located at lower pH values for the salt-containing acetate and citrate formulations than the maxima of their counterparts without salt. Contrary, the absence or presence of salt has only little impact on stability in the phosphate formulations for both IgG1 and IgG2 antibodies. With the data available from both heat- and agitation-induced degradation propensity, the correlation plot of percent monomer after 2 weeks of incubation at 40°C versus T_h values, obtained for each formulation from the midpoint of the lowest temperature transition from the first derivative of the fluorescence signal over a temperature range from 20°C to 95°C, is shown in Fig. 5.13. It is evident that a T_h of 50°C represents a threshold for monomeric antibody stability. Formulations with a T_h higher than 50°C have a monomeric antibody content of close to 90–95%, whereas formulations with a T_h below 45°C are highly degraded. Therefore it seems that the closer the unfolding temperature is to the incubation temperature, the higher the aggregation level become; a result that has direct implication on the selection of the final formulation with properties that provide thermal and conformational stability. In addition, it demonstrates the effectiveness of integrating automated sample preparation, high-throughput analytics, and statistical data analysis in evaluating formulation factors by a robust multivariate correlation analysis to develop a prediction model based on correlation analysis that helps to identify formulations with optimized stability properties. Basically, the analysis of high-throughput data provided a clear understanding and control of formulation stability.

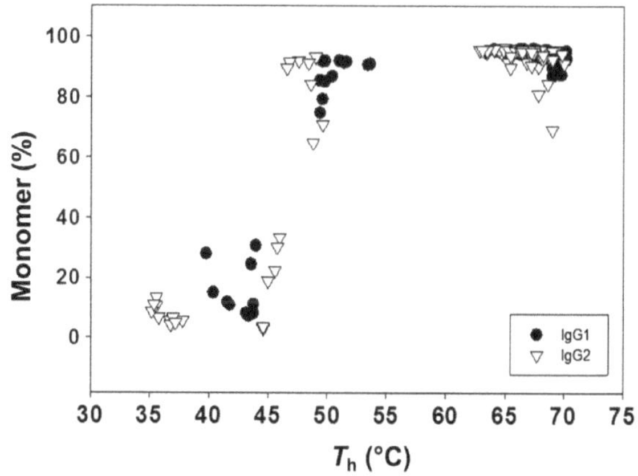

Figure 5.13 Correlation plot of percent monomer (from SE-UPLC data) versus T_h (from DSF data). SE-UPLC results were obtained after incubation of IgG1 (filled circles) and IgG2 (triangles) formulation samples for 2 weeks at 40°C.
Source: From L. Alekseychyk, C. Su, G.W. Becker, M.J. Treuheit, V.I. Razinkov, High-throughput screening and stability optimization of anti-streptavidin IgG1 and IgG2 formulations, J. Biomol. Screen. 19 (9) (2014) 1290–1301, Figure 2.

The construction of a reliable prediction model requires a very careful analysis of errors. In addition to the evaluation of actual versus predicted values, this can be achieved by residual analysis. The distribution of residuals should be randomly placed for all formulation conditions. Generally, the predicted values should be considered as directional rather than as absolutes for stability evaluation. Depending on the goodness of the fit, such evaluation can be more or less accurate. Also, statistical significance should not be confused with practical significance that is determined by actual experiments at relevant study conditions. For example, a change of 0.2% in percent monomer can be statistically significant by data analysis, but a 0.2% change in percent monomer may well be within the error of the analytical assay used for the measurement.

Although these works present examples for the development of an optimized formulation space, the optimization is based on a limited number of response factors. It is a reality in the formulation development laboratories of the biopharmaceutical industry that the number of variables and responses that are investigated in stability studies are generally much higher. In those cases where the experimental design needs to be more complex, the practicability of executing the large number of experimental analyses in a reasonable time frame is particularly depending on high-throughput methodologies and automation. Additionally, the interpretation of large data sets generated from these multivariate studies is very difficult not only because of the large number of data points but mainly because of the high dimensionality of the data. For example, the biophysical characterization of a protein's structural properties as a function of formulation composition, pH, and protein concentration can be performed by a number of different assays such as circular dichroism, intrinsic (tryptophan) and extrinsic fluorescence spectroscopy, light scattering, and DSC measurements. Each of these methods measures only one or two variables (dimensions) of a protein molecule's conformational properties. In many cases the results obtained by one technique may seem to contradict the results of another method. To understand multivariate relationships, systematic statistical analysis is necessary for constructing appropriate correlation models that help identify the significant correlations between the assessed structural properties and the conditions the protein was exposed to. An excellent example of such a methodology was described by Maddux et al., who applied multidimensional methods to formulation screening [16]. The applied methodology employed different statistical tools such as singular value decomposition and principal components analysis to decrease dimensionality of the data and make the results visibly more intuitive and interpretable for identifying the most stable formulation. To visualize the results of multiple experiments, the Empirical Phase Diagram (EPD) [17,18] is a method that has been used in many formulation studies including studies of vaccines [19], toxins [20], and antibodies [21]. In one example, the peptide pramlintide was characterized using a combination of circular dichroism, intrinsic fluorescence, second-derivative UV absorbance spectroscopy, as well as optical density measurements, as a function of pH, temperature, and peptide concentration [22]. The results from these assays were compiled into a normalized experimental data set and portrayed as a vector in an n-dimensional vector space of independent variables such as temperature, pH, and peptide concentration. All the individual vectors for

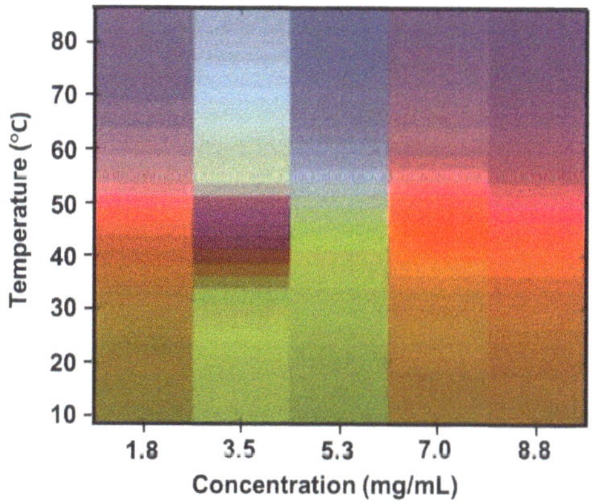

Figure 5.14 Empirical phase diagrams (EPDs) of pramlintide at low and high concentration and concentration dependence at pH 4. Low concentrations are represented as EPD of UV absorbance peak shift, OD_{350}, and fluorescence peak shift, and intensity data at pH 4 as a function of peptide concentration.
Source: From A. Nonoyama, J.S. Laurence, L. Garriques, H. Qi, T. Le, C.R. Middaugh, A biophysical characterization of the peptide drug pramlintide (AC137) using empirical phase diagrams, J. Pharm. Sci. 97 (7) (2008) 2552–2567, Figure 9.

each characterization assay created a density matrix and the eigenvalues and eigenvectors were calculated for the density matrix. The three components corresponding to the three largest eigenvalues were selected and a phase diagram was generated employing an arbitrary RGB (red/green/blue) color scheme to represent the three largest contributions to the final vectors. In Fig. 5.14 the temperature versus peptide concentration EPD is shown for the concentration dependence of pramlintide behavior at pH 4 as it was examined by UV absorbance spectroscopy, OD_{350} measurements, and fluorescence spectroscopy data. At the three highest peptide concentrations, the color transition from lower to higher temperatures was found to be relatively smooth. At 1.8 and 3.5 mg/mL, however, the small deviations in the OD_{350} experiments appeared as phases between 40°C and 50°C. The visible differences in color between particular concentrations could be attributed to the small differences in the absolute wavelength values of the fluorescence peak positions.

In another example by the same group, two mAbs were characterized at high protein concentrations as a function of temperature [23]. Spectroscopic techniques such as fluorescence, second-derivative UV absorbance, and circular dichroism spectroscopy were used to evaluate structural changes as a function of temperature and protein concentration. The data are summarized in form of temperature versus protein concentration EPDs (Fig. 5.15) for two monoclonal antibodies (mAb 1 and mAb 2). The phase diagram shown for mAb 1 (Fig. 5.15A) indicates a similar conformational state over the entire protein concentration range at temperatures $< 50°C$. At low protein concentrations, the phase changes correspond to a slightly unfolded and aggregated state at temperatures $> 65°C$. For higher protein concentrations, the empirical phases at higher temperatures have different colors and correspond to unfolded, aggregated,

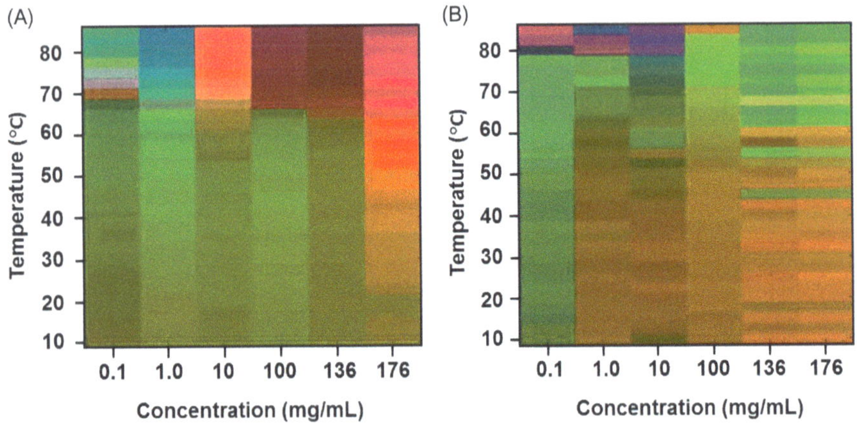

Figure 5.15 (A) Empirical phase diagram (EPD) of mAb 1 on a temperature versus concentration axis. Each temperature/concentration point on the diagram is constructed from data pertaining to fluorescence emission λ_{max}, OD_{350}, second-derivative UV absorbance peak positions of Phe, Tyr, and Trp, and molar ellipticity. (B) EPD of mAb 2 on a temperature versus concentration axis. Each temperature/concentration point on the diagram is constructed from data pertaining to fluorescence emission λ_{max}, OD_{350}, second-derivative UV absorbance peak positions of Phe, Tyr, and Trp, and molar ellipticity.
Source: From N. Harn, C. Allan, C. Oliver, C.R. Middaugh, Highly concentrated monoclonal antibody solutions: direct analysis of physical structure and thermal stability. J. Pharm. Sci. 96 (3) (2007) 532–546, Figure 10.

and precipitated conformational states. The phase diagram for mAb 2 (Fig. 5.15B) does not represent large structural changes. They are produced by differences in the biophysical results that are exaggerated by the normalization process across the RGB color scale. However, the phase boundaries are clear and visible enough to compare data between the mAb 1 and mAb 2 molecules at high protein concentrations. Therefore, EPD methods can be very useful for creating formulation stability profiles at different stages of drug development.

To compare the combined results of biophysical characterization data obtained by different techniques, the comparative signature diagram has been proposed by Iyer et al. [24]. This methodology compares data sets from different biophysical techniques that fingerprint the secondary, tertiary, and quaternary structures of a protein molecule and displays statistically significant differences in these data sets. Two proteins in various formulations were compared and several statistical tools were applied and evaluated to point out the most significant differences in protein and formulation signatures. High-throughput measurements and correlation analysis to evaluate conformational stability have been used in the study of 77 antibodies in the work by researchers from Pfizer [25]. In their work both intrinsic and extrinsic fluorescence-based assays were used to screen the thermal and pH dependent stability of antibody formulations. No correlation could be found between pH and thermal stability data. A machine-learning approach, using the large data set that was generated to predict biophysical properties from the primary sequence alone, was successful in predicting pH dependent mAb stability. The methodology of design of experiments (DOE) has been used to evaluate the stability and particle properties of antibody formulations by the means of a spray drying process [26]. The investigated formulations contained mannitol and trehalose as stabilizers at different ratios. A Plackett–Burman factorial design was used to identify the main factors of formulation and process, which significantly influenced the responses. The spray drying parameters were inlet temperature, air flow rate, solution concentration, liquid feed rate, and aspiration percent. The responses that were evaluated in the design were spray drying yield, particle size, size distribution, moisture content, and protein stability. SE-HPLC and FTIR were used to measure the amount of monomer and degree of secondary structure, respectively. The results of this study indicated that the atomization flow rate and type of sugar with various ratios was able to efficiently enhance particle properties.

A critical step in the experimental design of formulation studies is the selection of an adequately large number of replicates. The number of replicated experiments should be statistically sufficient to enable the detection of significant difference between experimental conditions if such differences exist. Although replicates can significantly increase the number of samples and experiments and therefore take more time to complete, they bear the benefit of enabling the detection of meaningful differences between experimental conditions. The cost of adding replicates is particularly high for studies that address binary response variables (e.g., "yes"/"no") over those with quantitative response variables such as formulation stability studies designed for the detection of particles. The response variable for these type of particle detection studies is either present (yes) or absent (no). To balance the practicality of executing studies with large sample sizes and the risk of conducting statistically underpowered studies that are not able to estimate the effects of interactions between significant factors, the application of Formal Experimental Design [27] may lead to substantial time and cost savings over one-factor-at-a-time experimentation because of the inherent property of "hidden replication" [28]. Hence, an appropriate designed experimental plan may assist in obtaining meaningful results in a less costly and time consuming way.

The methodology of artificial neural network (ANN) is another statistical analysis and prediction approach that has been applied in the field of pharmaceutical formulation development. ANN can be used as a multiobjective simultaneous optimization technique in cases when several responses relating to stability, efficacy, and safety must be optimized simultaneously [29]. The major advantage of this method is a more accurate estimation of the optimal formulation space when traditional response surface methodologies are generating satisfactory results. There is low bias in the ANN methodology and it can be applied to a wide range of formulation conditions without prior knowledge of specific protein stability properties. Another interesting application of ANN was found in the inspection of foreign particles in injection liquids. Pulse-coupled neural network, a modified ANN algorithm, was used in an automatic inspection machine to monitor the formation of visible particles in injection liquids [30] based on the continuity and smoothness of the particles' moving traces, which distinguishes particles in solution from static scratches and spots on the surface of vials.

Many modern data analysis techniques have been developed to serve high-throughput screening studies that use cell-based assays or other activity-based techniques to discover a "hit" in data sets generated from large numbers of samples. There are numerous reviews published on this topic. Although they may need some modifications, all these techniques can be also applied to the analysis of formulation screening data. It is quite common to assume for high-throughput screening data that they follow a normal distribution or are in compliance with the central limit theorem that states that the arithmetic mean of the values will be approximately normally distributed [31]. To achieve a more symmetric distribution around the mean data value, data transformation can be applied to the data during preprocessing. It may be useful to present relationships between variables in a more linear manner. The dependence of viscosity on protein concentration may be better presented by logarithmic transformation because, as described previously [7], viscosity increases sharply for formulations with higher protein concentrations. Hence, the presence of outliers can be a serious problem in the analysis of high-throughput data. Deviations from the normal distribution caused by the presence of outliers decreases the quality of regression models and overall prediction. In many cases the analysis of outliers is necessary to distinguish possible instrument errors from meaningful effects induced by formulation conditions. To remove outlier effects from data analyses, two main statistical approaches are commonly used: the classical and the robust method. In the classical method, outliers can be replaced or removed by calculating a truncated mean by discarding a certain percentage of the lowest and highest values and then computing the mean of the remaining values. The robust method can be described as the median absolute deviation from median, commonly shortened to the median absolute deviation. It is the median of the set comprising the absolute values of the differences between the median and each data point and is effectively used instead of mean and standard deviation to minimize the effect of outliers [32,33]. More recently, the methods of robust statistics have become a promising approach in the analysis of high-throughput data because of their reduced sensitivity to outliers. In high-throughput screening, even after consideration of all factors during method optimization, some variability in raw data is expected to remain such as random, unpredictable assay variability, which can be separated from the systematic errors caused by known factors like instrumental malfunction or failure. For many plate-based assays it is helpful to normalize the data within each plate to make data comparison across the plates possible. Two main methods are commonly used to normalize high-throughput data. One is a control-based approach, in which positive and negative controls are placed on the same plate where the samples are located. However, as in the analysis high or low variability in the control wells does not properly represent the variability in the sample wells, the outliers and biases related to control wells may affect the highest and lowest limits of the measurements [31,34]. The other method is a noncontrol-based normalization approach and is a better choice for gaining an overall understanding of a data distribution when only a few formulation conditions result in a significant output effect. In this method, most of the samples are assumed to have an insignificant response in order to serve as "negative controls," with the caveat that this approach may be misleading in cases when most of the wells on a screening plate express in fact a significant response. Therefore, experimentation-based normalization is preferred in screening studies where the effect of formulation factors is clustered within the constraints of particular plates and each plate is analyzed as a part of an all-plates screen. A plate-based approach can correct systematic errors specific to a plate without any distortion of the results obtained on other plates.

In addition to random fluctuations during method execution, systematic errors can occur because of instrumental errors and malfunction. A prominent example of a systematic error is the spatial irregularities of incubation conditions caused by plate geometry. The temperature can be distributed non-uniformly across different wells or vials on a plate and can result in a so-called "edge effect", which means that samples in wells on the edge of a plate experience a different temperature and therefore produce results that are different from results derived from samples located in wells in the middle of a plate. Depending on the position on a plate, column- or row-related effects may be observed. Inaccurate sample distribution by liquid-handling systems to the plate might also cause erroneous spatial pattern. Experiment-depending patterns should be verified by visual inspection and/or by measurements of such parameters as volume for each well. Some of the systematic issues can be corrected during the validation stage. There are also a number of methods to minimize the patterns of errors during the analysis of high-throughput data. The most common methods include: B-score, BZ-score, median polish, diffusion-state model, background correction, well-correction, etc.

The number of data points and sample size, as well as information about protein solubility and structural stability is very important for the accuracy of prediction. There are various prediction methods available for data analysis with different levels of bias and variance [35,36]. High-bias and low-variance methods include linear regression, discriminant analysis, partial least squares, and many others. These techniques are more stable and very well suited for formulation study designs that produce data points for a large number of response variables. Computationally these methods require fewer resources than low-bias techniques. However, they lack the ability to model complex, nonlinear relationships between formulation factors and response variables, but can be used for high-throughput robustness studies to build good prediction models because of a high probability of linear correlations between tested characteristics within a narrow range of formulation variables. Small increments of formulation factors are useful for mapping out a formulation space to determine the boundaries of stability inside which the changes in response variables are statistically insignificant. Comparability studies for the assessment of biosimilars are another example for the application of high-bias methods. More exploratory analyses using low-bias and high-variance methods include predictive models such as the above-mentioned neural networks, support vector machines, and k-Nearest Neighbors (k-NN). These models can be used for complex formulation screening studies of candidates with unknown or little known properties. Formulation screening studies of modalities with not well-characterized and understood properties and correlations between formulation factors and response variables are better modeled with low-bias prediction models, in which nonlinear correlations and interactions between factors are more probable. With both methods, the high-bias and low-bias models, the number of experimental data points or sample size can significantly reduce variance and improve the mean squared error, with the caveat that with an increasing number of measurements the computation time is usually increasing as well. For example, to analyze the sedimentation velocity data obtained by analytical ultracentrifugation (AUC), the absorbance measurements during the sedimentation time along the cell containing the protein can be performed at a resolution of either 100 or 300 data points. The model is the numerical fit of the Lamm equation, which describes the sedimentation and diffusion of a solute under ultracentrifugation [37]. At low resolution (i.e., 100 data points) the calculation takes about 20 minutes on a typical personal computer (c.2010), but can take up to several hours when the calculation is performed with a high-resolution data set (i.e., 300 data points). Along those lines, to improve model performance, drug development and particularly formulation development has been increasingly moving toward stability and comparability studies that utilize multidimensional measurements to collect an expanded number of meaningful attributes, rather than just expanding the number of data points. However, this approach runs the risk of including non-informative data that can greatly reduce model accuracy and efficiency. Therefore, to accurately model protein stability in a formulation or a variety of formulations over a long period of time at a recommended storage temperature (e.g., 2–8°C), it is important to include measurements that properly represent the attributes relevant at that storage condition. For example, at ambient temperatures and below, the measurement of the colloidal stability of the native conformation of a protein is in most cases more predictable of long-term stability than measurements of the conformational stability that is a more appropriate measure for a protein's stability at elevated storage and handling temperatures. Also, chemical stability is usually not a critical factor at low temperatures. Consequently, measurements of chemical modifications may be costly and require additional resources without improving the quality of the prediction model. Data, generated by high-throughput analyses, may assist in the ability to discover unique correlations and interactions that may not become available by traditional analysis. For example, the screening of excipients in a low-throughput format is usually conducted by individually testing formulations containing one excipient at a time. Expanding the number of samples would allow the screening of excipient mixtures and formulations with different excipient ratios. Some of those excipient combinations and ratios may improve stability and statistical modeling accuracy for predicting protein–excipient interactions, as well as their significance.

5.3 Closing words

In addition to planning and executing studies for formulation development that are appropriately designed for statistical analysis, the data analysis portion of an experiment is the most critical step in obtaining meaningful outcomes from complex, multivariate formulation studies. Whether an experiment or study is producing meaningful and valuable results for determining the formulation design space for a protein drug product depends on the experimental design and the choice of conditions and formulation components that are included as variable and distinguishing factors, as well as the response factors that are monitored and recorded.

To this end, after obtaining experimental data, possible correlations and interactions between responses and conditions should be established. For defining a formulation design space, the appropriate factors representing the formulation and conditions the formulations is exposed to need to be included in the experimental design and relevant response factors need to be recorded for analysis. Factors describing the formulation include factors like buffer type, pH, excipient, and surfactants. Factors describing external conditions include temperature, humidity, time, and different container types such as vials, syringes, or devices. Therefore, due to this complexity of formulation components, conditions, and response factors, the data generated by formulation studies require multivariate analysis to characterize and describe the design space of a given formulation.

References

[1] C. Kalonia, O.S. Kumru, J.H. Kim, C.R. Middaugh, D.B. Volkin, Radar chart array analysis to visualize effects of formulation variables on IgG1 particle formation as measured by multiple analytical techniques, J. Pharm. Sci. 102 (12) (2013) 4256–4267.

[2] M. Boulet-Audet, B. Byrne, S.G. Kazarian, High-throughput thermal stability analysis of a monoclonal antibody by ATR-FTIR spectroscopic imaging, Anal. Chem. 86 (19) (2014) 9786–9793.

[3] US Food and Drug Administration. Guidance for industry. Pharmaceutical cGMPs for the 21st Century—A Risk-Based Approach Final Report. Rockville, MD, September 2004.

[4] A.S. Rathore, H. Winkle, Quality by design for biopharmaceuticals, Nat. Biotechnol. 27 (2009) 26–34.

[5] M.R. Stoner, N. Fischer, L. Nixon, S. Buckel, M. Benke, F. Austin, et al., Protein–solute interactions affect the outcome of ultrafiltration/diafiltration operations, J. Pharm. Sci. 93 (9) (2004) 2332–2342.

[6] C. Harinarayan, K. Skidmore, Y. Kao, A.L. Zydney, R. Van Reis, Small molecule clearance in ultrafiltration/diafiltration in relation to protein interactions: study of citrate binding to a Fab, Biotechnol. Bioeng. 102 (6) (2009) 1718–1722.

[7] W.F. Smith, Experimental Design for Formulation, ASA-SIAM Series on Statistics and Applied Probability, SIAM, Philadelphia, 2005, ASA, Alexandria, VA.

[8] A.O. Grillo, M. Kane, N. Penn, M. Perkins, Characterizing the formulation design space, BioPharm. Int. 23 (3) (2010) 30.

[9] F. He, C.E. Woods, E. Trilisky, K.M. Bower, J.R. Litowski, B.A. Kerwin, et al., Screening of monoclonal antibody formulations based on high-throughput thermostability and viscosity measurements: design of experiment and statistical analysis, J. Pharm. Sci. 100 (4) (2011) 1330–1340.

[10] A. Saluja, A.V. Badkar, D.L. Zeng, S. Nema, D.S. Kalonia, Ultrasonic storage modulus as a novel parameter for analyzing protein-protein interactions in high protein concentration solutions: correlation with static and dynamic light scattering measurements, Biophys. J. 92 (1) (2007) 234–244.

[11] J.R. Livingstone, R.S. Spolar, M.T. Record, Jr, Contribution to the thermodynamics of protein folding from the reduction in water-accessible nonpolar surface area, Biochemistry 30 (17) (1991) 4237–4244.

[12] F. He, S. Hogan, R.F. Latypov, L.O. Narhi, V.I. Razinkov, High throughput thermostability screening of monoclonal antibody formulations, J. Pharm. Sci. 99 (4) (2010) 1707–1720.

[13] F. He, G.W. Becker, J.R. Litowski, L.O. Narhi, D.N. Brems, V.I. Razinkov, High-throughput dynamic light scattering method for measuring viscosity of concentrated protein solutions, Anal. Biochem. 399 (1) (2010) 141–143.

[14] F. He, C.E. Woods, G.W. Becker, L.O. Narhi, V.I. Razinkov, High-throughput assessment of thermal and colloidal stability parameters for monoclonal antibody formulations, J. Pharm. Sci. 100 (12) (2011) 5126–5141.

[15] L. Alekseychyk, C. Su, G.W. Becker, M.J. Treuheit, V.I. Razinkov, High-throughput screening and stability optimization of anti-streptavidin IgG1 and IgG2 formulations, J. Biomol. Screen. 19 (9) (2014) 1290–1301.

[16] N.R. Maddux, S.B. Joshi, D.B. Volkin, J.P. Ralston, C.R. Middaugh, Multidimensional methods for the formulation of biopharmaceuticals and vaccines, J. Pharm. Sci. 100 (10) (2011) 4171–4197.

[17] L.A. Kueltzo, B. Ersoy, J.P. Ralston, C.R. Middaugh, Derivative absorbance spectroscopy and protein phase diagrams as tools for comprehensive protein characterization: a bGCSF case study, J. Pharm. Sci. 92 (9) (2003) 1805–1820.

[18] S.B. Joshi, A. Bhambhani, Y. Zeng, C.R. Middaugh, An empirical phase diagram–high-throughput screening approach to the characterization and formulation of biopharmaceuticals: Formulation and Process Development Strategies for Manufacturing Biopharmaceuticals, Wiley, Hoboken, NJ, (2010) 173–205.

[19] Y. Zeng, H. Fan, G. Chiueh, B. Pham, R. Martin, D. Lechuga-Ballesteros, et al., Towards development of stable formulations of a live attenuated bacterial vaccine, Hum. Vaccin. 5 (5) (2009) 322–331.

[20] M.S. Salnikova, S.B. Joshi, J.H. Rytting, M. Warny, C.R. Middaugh, Physical characterization of *Clostridium difficile* toxins and toxoids: effect of the formaldehyde crosslinking on thermal stability, J. Pharm. Sci. 97 (9) (2008) 3735–3752.

[21] A. Bhambhani, J.M. Kissmann, S.B. Joshi, D.B. Volkin, R.S. Kashi, C.R. Middaugh, Formulation design and high-throughput excipient selection based on structural integrity and conformational stability of dilute and highly concentrated IgG1 monoclonal antibody solutions, J. Pharm. Sci. 101 (3) (2012) 1120–1135.

[22] A. Nonoyama, J.S. Laurence, L. Garriques, H. Qi, T. Le, C.R. Middaugh, A biophysical characterization of the peptide drug pramlintide (AC137) using empirical phase diagrams, J. Pharm. Sci. 97 (7) (2008) 2552–2567.

[23] N. Harn, C. Allan, C. Oliver, C.R. Middaugh, Highly concentrated monoclonal antibody solutions: direct analysis of physical structure and thermal stability, J. Pharm. Sci. 96 (3) (2007) 532–546.

[24] V. Iyer, N. Maddux, L. Hu, W. Cheng, A.K. Youssef, G. Winter, et al., Comparative signature diagrams to evaluate biophysical data for differences in protein structure across various formulations, J. Pharm. Sci. 102 (1) (2013) 43–51.

[25] A.C. King, M. Woods, W. Liu, Z. Lu, D. Gill, M.R. Krebs, High-throughput measurement, correlation analysis, and machine-learning predictions for pH and thermal stabilities of Pfizer-generated antibodies, Protein Sci. 20 (9) (2011) 1546–1557.

[26] V. Ramezani, A. Vatanara, A. Rouholamini Najafabadi, K. Gilani, M. Nabi-Meybodi, Screening and evaluation of variables in the formation of antibody particles by spray drying, Powder Technol. 233 (2013) 341–346.

[27] Q8 Pharmaceutical Development (2006). International Conference on Harmonisation of Technical Requirements for Registration of Pharmaceuticals for Human Use (ICH). <http://www.fda.gov/downloads/RegulatoryInformation/Guidances/ucm128029.pdf>.

[28] K.M. Bower, A. Germansderfer, B.A. Kerwin, G.R. Kleemann, J.R. Litowski, Designed experiments with binary responses, J. Pharm. Sci. 100 (11) (2011) 5078–5079.

[29] K. Takayama, M. Fujikawa, Y. Obata, M. Morishita, Neural network based optimization of drug formulations, Adv. Drug Deliv. Rev. 55 (9) (2003) 1217–1231.
[30] J. Ge, Y. Wang, B. Zhou, H. Zhang, Intelligent foreign particle inspection machine for injection liquid examination based on modified pulse-coupled neural networks, Sensors 9 (5) (2009) 3386–3404.
[31] M. Entzeroth, H. Flotow, P. Condron, Overview of high-throughput screening, Curr. Protoc. Pharmacol. (2009) 9.4.1–9.4.23.
[32] I. Coma, J. Herranz, J. Martin, Statistics and decision making in high throughput screening, in: W.P. Janzen, P. Bernasconi, (Eds.), High Throughput Screening, Methods in Molecular Biology, Methods and Protocols, Humana Press, New York, NY, 2009, pp. 69–106. ISBN 9781603272575.
[33] P.J. Huber, Robust Statistics, Springer, Berlin Heidelberg, 2011,1248–1251.
[34] S.A. Sundberg, High throughput and ultra-high-throughput screening: solution-and cell-based approaches, Curr. Opin. Biotechnol. 11 (1) (2000) 47–53.
[35] C. Brideau, B. Gunter, B. Pikounis, A. Liaw, Improved statistical methods for hit selection in high-throughput screening, J. Biomol. Screen. 8 (6) (2003) 634–647.
[36] M. Kuhn, K. Johnson, Applied Predictive Modeling, Springer, New York, NY, 2013,6192
[37] J. Lebowitz, M.S. Lewis, P. Schuck, Modern analytical ultracentrifugation in protein science: a tutorial review, Protein Sci. 11 (9) (2002) 2067–2079.

Index

Note: Page numbers followed by "*f*" and "*t*" refer to figures and tables, respectively.

FSC
www.fsc.org
MIX
Papier | Fördert
gute Waldnutzung
FSC® C083411

Kolibri 360 GmbH
Ferdinand-Jühlke-Straße 7
99095 Erfurt, Deutschland
produktsicherheit@kolibri360.de